KU-203-186

FIGHTING THE SILENT KILLER

How Men and Women Can Prevent and Cope with Heart Disease Today

Dr. Peter F. Cohn
Dr. Joan K. Cohn

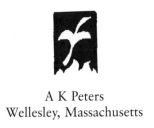

A K Peters
Wellesley, Massachusetts

Editorial, Sales, and Customer Service Office
A K Peters, Ltd.
289 Linden Street
Wellesley, MA 02181

Copyright © 1993 by AK Peters, Ltd.

All rights reserved. No part of the material protected by this copyright notice may be reproduced or utilized in any form, electronic or mechanical, including photocopying, recording, or by any information storage and retrieval system, without written permission from the copyright owner.

Portions of this publication were previously published in Heart Talk: Preventing and Coping with Silent and Painful Heart Disease by Dr. Peter F. Cohn and Dr. Joan K. Cohn, Harcourt Brace Jovanovich, Inc., 1987.

Library of Congress Cataloging-in-Publication Data

Cohn, Peter F., 1939–
    Fighting the Silent Killer: How Men and Women Can Prevent and Cope With Heart Disease Today
        p.   cm.
    Includes bibliographical references.
    ISBN 0-15-139830-5 : ISBN 1-56881-021-0
    1. Coronary heart disease—Popular works. 2. Coronary heart disease—Prevention.
I. Cohn, Joan K. II. Cohn, Peter F., 1939– Heart Talk. III. Title.
RC685.C6C585 1993
616.1'23—dc20   93-31115
                                                                                  CIP

Printed in the United States of America
97 96 95 94 93   10 9 8 7 6 5 4 3 2 1

This book is dedicated to our parents
and to our children

Contents

Preface

When we originally conceived the idea for this book in 1986 we were concerned that few Americans were sufficiently aware of the latest developments in preventing and treating heart disease.* In 1987, we published *Heart Talk: Preventing and Coping With Silent and Painful Heart Disease* to address these issues. In the last six years, the need for up-to-date awareness of heart disease has not diminished, but rather new areas have arisen which need to be explored and understood by the lay public. Despite the continuing decline in deaths due to heart disease, it still remains our number one killer, far exceeding the number of deaths caused by cancer and AIDS combined.

There is no question that in the last two decades Americans have become increasingly health conscious. Their diets contain appreciably less fat and cholesterol, they have reduced or eliminated cigarette smoking, and they exercise more. Adopting these healthful habits has dramatically reversed the death rate from cardiovascular causes, especially heart attacks. However heart disease is still the nation's number one killer, and more needs to be done.

Ironically, as the general trend towards fewer deaths from cardiovascular disease has become apparent, so has the recognition of a new aspect of heart disease. This new phenomenon is "silent" heart disease. It is becoming increasingly obvious to physicians—and to the lay public as well—that serious heart

---

* Throughout this book, *heart disease* will refer to *coronary* heart disease, the type of heart disease resulting from blockages in blood supply to the heart muscle itself. Other, less common, forms of heart disease will be mentioned only briefly.

disease can exist in the absence of symptoms. The first manifestation of disease can be catastrophic: death or a major heart attack with irreversible destruction of large amounts of heart muscle. *All of this can occur without warning.* There is also evidence that people who have suffered a heart attack and survived and are apparently healthy may also be experiencing episodes of painless damage to the heart. Finally, additional information shows that many patients whose cardiac pain is apparently well-controlled with medicines or surgery are still experiencing episodes of heart disease, but without pain.

Because millions of people in the United States and other Western societies suffer from silent heart disease, it is emerging as a major public health problem. The idea that we must detect and treat both painful and silent episodes of heart damage is a new and exciting one in cardiovascular medicine today. It means that doctors must not only listen to what the patient's mouth says, but what the patient's heart says. This "heart talk" is not just for doctors. Lessons learned from listening to the heart can be useful to all of us. That is why we wrote this book—to focus attention on new advances in the battle against heart disease by disclosing as much as is known about painful and silent heart disease. How does silent disease relate to symptomatic heart disease? What are the common features of both types of heart disease? How is heart disease related to diet, exercise, and stress? Is there a "mind-body connection" with heart disease? How does silent heart disease—because it lacks an element of warning—pose special problems in detection and treatment? In other words, how do we fight this silent killer?

There are additional questions about the problem of women and heart disease. Is it really a worse problem than breast cancer? Why do some women seem protected until menopause and not others? What is the importance of an oat bran diet? Of Vitamin E? Then, too, there are the exciting new developments with "clot-busters" for heart attacks and "roto-rooters" for shelling out those fatty deposits that block the blood supply to the heart.

Even though heart disease is highly unpredictable, the "answers" we provide are factual and, we hope, encouraging. For example, some readers will have a greater likelihood of developing coronary artery disease because they are male, and their fathers, grandfathers, and/or uncles developed heart disease when they were young (under 55). Because of this, they may feel that their fate is sealed and there is nothing they can do. On the contrary, knowing that heart disease is prevalent in your family should serve as a red flag. It should make you take notice, perhaps make you angry, but, most of all, warn you *to do something about it*. Even though your genes may predispose you to coronary artery disease, if you can "correct" certain factors (such as high blood pressure and cigarette smoking), your chances for good health will be improved immeasurably.

To provide our readers with helpful guidelines, including advice about exercise and diets, we have drawn from our own experiences at the State University of New York Health Sciences Center at Stony Brook (one of the international centers for research in this subject) as well as from the experiences of other experts from around the world. We welcome your comments. Our address is the Cardiology Division, SUNY Health Sciences Center, Stony Brook, New York 11794–8171.

Encouragement from friends in the United States and Europe was invaluable in the writing of this book. We would especially like to thank Marlene Landesman and Klaus and Alice Peters for assisting us with this update edition.

CHAPTER
1

A New Concept
in Heart Disease

Results of recent research in heart disease show that many episodes of heart disease are painless. The medical terms are *silent myocardial ischemia* (painless angina, in lay terms) and *silent, or unrecognized, myocardial infarction* (painless heart attacks). Perhaps the most frightening aspect of silent heart disease is that it can be undetected until the affected individual dies suddenly and unexpectedly. This happens over a thousand times a week in the United States.

———————

There is a killer at loose in our country. Not a killer with a gun or a knife, but one whose weapons are the cigarette and the beefsteak. The killer is heart disease—but not just the painful type of heart disease the public has been taught to be aware of, the kind that is accompanied by crushing chest pains. The killer can also be silent. Heart disease does not have to be accompanied by pain—or any other symptoms, for that matter! That is why it is so important to be knowledgeable about both painful and *painless* episodes of heart disease. How can heart disease be prevented, detected and treated if so many episodes are painless?

These are questions that doctors are hearing more and more frequently from concerned patients who read and hear the term *silent heart disease* in newspapers, magazines, medical reports, and on the radio and television. The following two scenarios, both based closely on actual case histories, will help introduce the reader to this enigmatic subject.

Mr. Jones is in apparent good health. He is 50 years old, slightly overweight and has a one-pack-a-day smoking habit that he has tried to give up several times. One morning he kisses his wife and children goodbye, as he normally does, and hurries off to catch the commuter train to his office. He never returns. In fact, he gets no further than the railroad station. After hurrying up the steps, he suddenly collapses on the platform. Fellow passengers try to help. Station police arrive several minutes later but can feel no pulse in his wrist or neck. An ambulance crew arrives and attempts to resuscitate Mr. Jones, but 30 minutes of futile attempts at restoring a heartbeat convinces the crew that the situation is hopeless. The body is taken to the nearest hospital, where Mr. Jones is pronounced DOA (dead on arrival). Because no known illness had caused his demise, an autopsy is ordered by the county medical examiner and performed two days later.

When the pathologist doing the autopsy first sees Mr. Jones's heart, there are no obvious signs of a fatal disease. Only when the blade of the scalpel slits the outer lining of one of the heart's major blood vessels does the pathologist discover the cause of death. Instead of the clear central space he expected to find in the blood vessel, there is a hard, gritty substance with barely enough of a channel through its core to allow anything but the most minimal stream of blood. As the pathologist's exploration continues, he sees that *all* of Mr. Jones's major blood vessels on the surface of the heart have similar obstructions. Although the pathologist has seen this type of disease at many other autopsies, he is puzzled by the man's clinical history—or rather by the lack of it. How could Mr. Jones have died without any warning, without having had a previous heart attack, without even having transient episodes of chest pain? How was this possible, considering all the years that it must have taken for the deposits of cholesterol and other material to turn the normally soft, compliant blood vessels of the heart into hard, rigid and barely passable conduits?

There is no satisfactory answer that the pathologist can provide for these questions, and he knows from previous experience that his colleagues cannot either. All he is sure of is that the man is dead and that he will write "sudden cardiac death due to coronary atherosclerosis without preceeding symptoms" in his report to the medical examiner.

What happened to Mr. Jones happens over a thousand times a week in the United States! A previously healthy person dies suddenly and unexpectedly, and an autopsy later reveals severe heart disease. But there is another, less gruesome, type of scenario that also is part of the spectrum of silent heart disease.

Mr. Smith is also 50 years old and in apparent good health. He has also unsuccessfully tried to stop smoking. Fortunately, Mr. Smith, unlike Mr. Jones, has a physician who is concerned that he might be developing a heart condition. Not only is Mr. Smith a smoker, but he also has an abnormally high level of cholesterol in his blood. In addition, Mr. Smith's father had died at the age of 58 after experiencing a heart attack. For these reasons, Mr. Smith's physician recommends that he have a stress test.

To prepare Mr. Smith for the stress test, a technician attaches special adhesive patches (called electrodes) onto Mr. Smith's chest. A wire runs from each patch to a machine that records electrocardiographs. After having been wired to eight different sets of electrodes, Mr. Smith begins walking briskly on a treadmill while a cardiologist tracks his heartbeat as it is displayed on a green TV-like screen. The electrocardiographic signals follow one another in a normal, steady procession. Mr. Smith begins to perspire, but he does not feel pain or pressure in his chest or arm—the sensations that doctors know are telltale signs of a heart attack or the milder condition termed angina. Mr. Smith is not aware that the electrocardiographic signals are becoming abnormal; in particular, certain wave forms that should be horizontal are becoming more vertical. When his legs begin to grow weary, Mr. Smith knows he is ready to stop. The cardiologist readily agrees.

After stopping, Mr. Smith lies down on an examining table. His heart rate and blood pressure quickly return to their pre-exercise levels. But as the cardiologist explains, the abnormal waveforms that appeared in the electrical signals from the heart during the last few minutes of the test do not return to normal levels. These abnormalities persist on Mr. Smith's electrocardiogram for nearly 10 minutes after the stress test has been completed—a very unhealthy sign. Not only were these abnormalities visible on the monitor screen, they were also recorded on two-inch wide strips of lined paper specially calibrated into tiny boxes to allow easy measurement of different parts of the electrocardiographic signal. The cardiologist shows Mr. Smith one of the strips and comments that the abnormalities are of the same severity that are usually seen in patients with advanced heart disease. The cardiologist is concerned about these abnormalities and fears that they may indicate blockages in the coronary arteries. He wants Mr. Smith to stay in the hospital's coronary care unit and undergo a special X-ray procedure called coronary arteriography in the morning. After this procedure has been explained to him, Mr. Smith agrees to have it done.

In the morning, Mr. Smith receives a tranquilizer and mild sedative through an intravenous tube inserted in his arm. When he is drowsy, he is wheeled down the corridor to the cardiac catheterization laboratory. There technicians and nurses bustle about him in what seem random actions but are in fact part of a well-coordinated catheterization protocol that can evaluate two to three patients a day. As he lies on a special examining table, the hair near his groin is carefully shaved in preparation for the insertion of the catheters. This is necessary to keep the area as free of germs as possible. Mr. Smith has learned that to take X-ray pictures of the blood vessels of his heart (the coronary arteries), thin tubes called catheters will be introduced into a large artery at the top of the thigh and gently pushed up the aorta, the main blood channel of the body, to the area where the openings to the coronary arteries are located. (When opaque fluids are injected into the tubes, flow through the coronary arteries can be tracked). Once the doctors on the catheterization team have swabbed the skin over the thigh with an antiseptic solution, they deaden the skin by injecting an anesthetic drug and insert the first catheter. Mr. Smith is surprised at how swiftly the catheter is advanced to the openings of the coronary arteries. During the actual injection of the opaque substance into his coronary arteries, he is able to follow the path of these vessels on one of the TV monitors in the room. The procedure takes about an hour and, though somewhat uncomfortable, is not particularly painful.

In Mr. Smith's hospital room later that afternoon, the cardiologist draws diagrams to show him that two of his three major coronary arteries are severely diseased. He explains that while the amount of blood necessary to supply the muscle of the heart with life-supporting oxygen is about 125 ml every minute, Mr. Smith's damaged vessels can only supply 80 ml per minute. The result is a condition called *ischemia*: inadequate oxygenation of a part of the body due to reduced blood flow. This is what was suggested by the abnormal tracings on the electrocardiograms during the stress test. Mr. Smith learns that most people with ischemia of the heart complain of chest pain. When the ischemia is transient, the chest discomfort is called *angina*. When blood flow stops for more than 20 minutes, the affected parts of the heart die. This is termed an *infarction* and is known to most people as a heart attack. The cardiologist believes Mr. Smith may have been close to having a heart attack. Since he had no warning signs that his heart was being damaged, he might have done himself irreversible harm during some seemingly innocuous physical activity. Why he had no pain during the transient episodes of ischemia is a mystery, but Mr. Smith knows he is fortunate to have had the condition discovered.

Mr. Smith was lucky; he learned about his silent heart disease while there was still time to treat it. Unfortunately, Mr. Jones was not as lucky.

For many physicians, as well as members of the lay public, it had long been a given that serious heart disease was accompanied by one or more symptoms that help alert both the patient and his or her physician to the underlying problem. Today we know this is not true. In fact, there is increasing evidence that quite the opposite is true: Many, if not most, of the episodes of heart damage due to coronary heart disease are painless.

These two scenarios have illustrated one aspect of silent heart disease: Damage occurs in otherwise healthy persons. There are other scenarios, discussed in subsequent chapters, in which patients with known heart disease (such as prior heart attacks) are apparently pain free but find that their disease is continuing in a silent form. In yet other patients, heart disease will consist of various combinations of painful and silent episodes. The common thread in all these situations is the occurrence of heart damage with or without symptoms. But how and why does the damage occur in the first place?

Coronary heart disease (or as many physicians prefer to call it, coronary artery disease) is characterized by the buildup of fatty deposits called plaques, made up largely of cholesterol, in the walls of the coronary arteries. These arteries are the main source of blood supply to the muscle cells of that unique pumping organ of the human body, the heart. This atherosclerotic process is described in detail in Chapter 4. At this point, it suffices to say that the net result of these fatty deposits is reduction of the internal opening of the arteries, which means a lower blood flow to the heart muscle that the blood vessel serves. Heart disease is the number one killer in the United States; more than five million people are being treated for it and nearly 700,000 per year die of it. This number is by far the lion's share of the nearly one million people a year who die of cardiovascular disease (most of the rest die from strokes). In the cases of Mr. Smith and Mr. Jones, we have seen what happens when heart cells, because of inadequate blood supply, do not get enough oxygen to meet their needs. Such ischemia occurs for varying amounts of time. If the ischemia is transitory and lasts no more than several minutes, it does *not* lead to irreversible damage of heart muscle. More prolonged deprivation leads to irreversible damage, a heart attack, and often death.

Having said all of this, let us ask an additional key question: Where does pain fit into all of this? Why do you have a silent heart attack?

Cardiac pain such as angina is no more than the *patient's awareness* of damage—transient or permanent—being done to the heart. It does not tell us how severe the underlying disease is. In fact, there are many instances of individuals complaining of severe chest pain attributed to the heart for whom a thorough workup, including coronary arteriography, reveals no structural abnormalities at all! Perhaps psychosomatic mechanisms are involved. These individuals have normal life spans despite their unnervingly "typical" complaints of cardiac disease! And, of course, as we have already seen in the Smith/Jones scenarios, pain can be totally absent in the presence of severe cardiac disease. This does not mean that pain should be ignored; what it does mean is pain is not a reliable marker of transient ischemia or even heart attacks. In the public's perception of heart disease, however, pain or related symptoms (chest pressure, jaw or arm pain) loom large as synonyms for problems in the body's circulatory pump.

Why do we perceive chest pain as being closely linked to heart disease? The history of medicine is one in which the patient's complaints and a physical examination are the keystones of the physician's assessment. This is not surprising in light of the paucity of sophisticated diagnostic instruments in pre-twentieth century medicine. Physicians had to rely on what the patient said rather than what they found on examination—they had no recourse to the technology that the modern clinician has. Consequently, the physician was not, and could not, be aware that parts of the heart were being slowly but methodically deprived of their vital oxygen supplies if the patient had no cardiac symptoms and if the physical examination was normal—as it often is in coronary artery disease (especially silent heart disease).

With the invention of monitoring devices that allow us to record the sequence of physiologic events when a region of the heart is deprived of its required oxygen supply, we now know that pain is at the end of the sequence of events—if pain occurs at all! Why is pain a variable feature? Simply put, we don't know. Some of the theories will be discussed in detail in subsequent chapters, but we do know that pain is an inconsistent feature, and the phenomenon of silent heart disease is a result of this variability.

The major components of silent heart disease—in addition to death—are *silent myocardial ischemia* (painless angina) and *silent myocardial infarctions* (painless heart attacks). As the following scenario illustrates, the latter is purely an electrocardiographic diagnosis. Mr. Brown has a normal electrocardiographic examination on June 1, 1984, during his routine physical examination. In his next annual physical examination—June 5, 1985—his electrocardiogram is clearly abnormal: A heart attack has occurred involving the front wall of the heart's major chamber, the left ventricle. Despite persistent questioning by his physician, Mr. Brown denies having had any episode of chest pain or pressure in the past year, or for that matter, any "indigestion" serious enough to make him think about consulting a physician. The infarction is called silent or painless, or, perhaps more accurately, unrecognized. In Framingham, Massachusetts, the site of the famous Framingham Heart Study that we will discuss in Chapter 2, a quarter of all heart attacks were unrecognized!

A common way of observing silent (painless) ischemia is during an exercise test, also called a stress test. This test is ideal for seeing whether or not physical exertion can bring on ischemia because it is done in a controlled setting with immediate medical attention available. The exercise test is usually performed with a treadmill device that moves at a slowly increasing speed and incline. This is what was used to detect silent heart disease in Mr. Smith. While the cardiac abnormalities are being observed on the electrocardiograph, the patient can be continually questioned by physicians about symptoms.

Silent ischemia can be categorized into three types. The first type involves persons who are totally asymptomatic; cardiac abnormalities are only detected by exercise testing or related procedures. The second type includes patients who have had a heart attack and demonstrate silent ischemia during their routine convalescent stress test. The third type have painful angina but continuous 24-hour electrocardiographic monitoring shows that they also have repeated episodes of silent ischemia. (Detection of silent ischemia in these three types of patients is discussed in detail in later chapters.) Thus, heart disease in some individuals may consist of only silent episodes, while in others it is a combination of painful and silent episodes in various proportions. It is the first type of patient who may well go on to sudden death or a massive heart attack before—if ever at all—complaining of angina. This is what happened to Mr. Jones. Mr. Smith was fortunate enough to be diagnosed before such an event.

CHAPTER

2

How Common Is Silent Heart Disease Compared to Painful Heart Disease?

There are probably at least one to two million middle-aged men in the United States with blockages in their coronary arteries who are unaware that they have heart disease. Another 50,000 persons per year are found to have silent heart disease after they have apparently recovered from a painful heart attack. In addition, two million of the four million patients with painful angina also have frequent episodes of silent myocardial ischemia. These episodes can be documented with the use of an electrocardiographic device worn continuously during the day and night (the ambulatory ECG, or Holter, monitor).

We noted in Chapter 1 that over one thousand apparently healthy people die each week with autopsy-proven evidence of severe heart disease. The question can then be asked: How many people are walking around with undetected disease, waiting for their catastrophe to occur?

To answer it simply, *the number of individuals affected by silent heart disease is so large that it immediately transforms what otherwise might have only been a subject of academic interest to that of a major public health problem, as well as a challenge to contemporary therapeutic principles in cardiology.* Such a sweeping statement is only credible if it can be supported by facts. In the remainder of the chapter, we will provide the reader with these facts.

What is the frequency of silent ischemia in persons like Mr. Smith who seem to be totally free of heart disease but who are found to have abnormal stress tests and then have coronary arteriography that confirms the diagnosis of coronary heart disease? As one might imagine, obtaining accurate information about such individuals in the general population is not easy. There are several reasons for this difficulty. First, a mechanism must be set up whereby large numbers of apparently healthy persons are screened for the presence of coronary heart disease. Individuals who are most suspected of having the disease, because of risk factors and abnormal performance on screening procedures like the stress test, can then be referred for coronary arteriography. Factories, large corporations and service organizations are all suitable targets for screening workers, but the costs of the screening procedure are prohibitive for many private hospitals. Without specific research grants, they do not have the resources for such a study. Therefore, government supported or controlled hospitals are particularly well suited for this type of data collection.

Another major problem is convincing individuals with abnormal screening tests to submit to coronary arteriography, a procedure with a small but definite amount of complications (i.e., a 1% risk of death, heart attack or stroke). Also, overnight hospitalization is usually required and the procedure itself— although not painful, as Mr. Smith found out—is certainly not pleasant. Nonetheless, there are some studies that do provide us with rough estimates of the frequency of silent ischemia. One of the most important was performed by Dr. Jan Erikssen and his colleagues in Oslo, Norway. They screened 2019 symptom-free office workers and found 50 (or 2.5%) had positive stress tests and abnormal coronary arteriograms.

A similar figure was arrived at by a group of U.S. Air Force physicians who were screening flight personnel as part of a study aimed at reducing serious flight accidents due to heart disease in crews of U.S. Air Force planes. Of the 3000 individuals who were screened initially, 90 had evidence of coronary artery disease on their arteriograms. In 78 of these 90, the disease was severe enough to warrant prolonged follow-up.

In contrast to these two large studies, Dr. Rene Langou and associates at Yale University examined 129 healthy industrial workers in a nearby New Haven plant. Of the 129, 13 (10%) were subsequently shown by coronary arteriography to have coronary heart disease and 12 of the 13 had a severe form of obstruction. Thus, in these studies we have frequency rates ranging from 2.5–10%. Nearly all the persons screened were men aged 30–60, which we will henceforth call "middle-aged" in order to make assumptions concerning the public at large.

Another way of studying the number of asymptomatic persons with severe coronary artery disease is to "work backwards." In other words, analyze autopsy results of persons who have died from trauma (such as car accidents) or non-cardiac diseases (such as cancer) and for whom there was no history of cardiac complaints during life. This is a less exact technique for several reasons. First, the history-taking is retrospective. A person might have had an episode suspicious of cardiac disease but not have told family, friends, or physicians. Second, the obstructions noted at autopsy where the blood vessels are collapsed (drained of fluid) may appear more severe than they were during life, when the vessel walls containing the fatty deposits were distended by fluid under normal blood pressures. Third, the obstructions, although sinister in appearance, might not have actually produced damage during life.

Given these limitations, we can now put into perspective the frequency of asymptomatic disease derived from such autopsy studies. In an extensive review, Drs. George Diamond and James Forrester of the Cedars-Sinai Hospital in Los Angeles, a major teaching hospital of the UCLA School of Medicine, found that 6.4% of middle-aged men without prior cardiac histories had autopsy evidence of coronary heart disease. This figure was less (2.4%) in middle-aged women, probably as a result of the protective action of female hormones prior to menopause. In the same report, they examined the frequency of coronary artery disease in persons without chest pain who were undergoing cardiac catheterization because of their abnormal electrocardiograms, stress tests, etc. For this group, the figure was 4%.

In summary, we would conclude that the frequency of this type of silent ischemia is probably under 5%. Assuming an average of 4%, this would mean that *1–2 million of the 30–40 million asymptomatic middle-aged men in this country are affected. Considering that we are treating between 5–6 million men and women of all ages for known coronary artery disease, this is a staggering figure.*

What about patients with other types of silent heart disease? For example: Mr. White has had a heart attack but appears to be recovering uneventfully. It is now commonplace to perform a not particularly strenuous ("low-level") exercise stress test 10–14 days after a heart attack, usually before the patient is discharged from the hospital. Mr. White has such a test and the results are clearly abnormal, although he has no pain. Imagine his surprise when his cardiologist tells Mr. White that while he might think he's fine, his heart is saying the opposite!

This is how many of the patients with this second type of silent ischemia are detected—by abnormalities on their post-heart-attack stress test. In addition, it is not uncommon for patients to have standard stress tests six months after the heart attack and then on a one-year or two-year basis. Other cases of silent disease are detected by these tests. Of the 500,000 or so heart attack victims who are hospitalized each year in the United States, about 400,000 leave the hospital alive. Of these 400,000 survivors, about 150,000 are still troubled by cardiac problems including angina, irregularities of the heart rhythm or heart failure (a buildup of fluid throughout the body because of weak pumping action by the heart). The other 250,000 patients are "uncomplicated" and eligible for stress tests. Most (150,000) will have normal (negative) tests. The remaining 100,000 will have abnormal tests and about half of these will not have pain with such tests. These 50,000 patients per year represent newly found cases of silent ischemia. Not all patients will remain asymptomatic. Many will go on to have recurrent heart attacks or develop angina again (or for the first time). The total number of persons in this category thus remains elusive, but it is substantial.

Some of the individuals with angina will experience frequent episodes of silent ischemia in addition to their regular, painful episodes. This is the third type of silent ischemia. All of these episodes—painful and painless—can be detected by a special type of cardiac monitoring. The story behind this procedure is a fascinating one. Developed by Dr. Norman Holter, an engineer, and reported in 1961, this revolutionary technique allows long-term (24–48 hours) electrocardiographic recordings to be made while an individual walks, works, rests, etc. These recordings were originally used for detection of heart rhythm irregularities, but more recently they have been used for detection of ischemic episodes. The attachment of the electrodes is similar to a stress test, but there are fewer of them, and they are all connected to a small "black box" device that is strapped to the patient's waist (described in more detail in Chapter 3).

In 1977, Drs. Steven Schang and Carl Pepine of the University of Florida used Holter monitoring to demonstrate that three or four episodes of silent ischemia occurred for every episode of painful ischmia. When these results first appeared in a medical journal, they were greeted with some degree of skepticism. As we noted previously, ischemia without pain is a difficult concept for many physicians to accept. In addition, technical problems in the Holter system itself led some to question the reliability of its electrocardiographic demonstration of ischemia. Several years earlier, similiar skepticism had greeted the reports of Drs. Dan Tzivoni and Shlomo Stern in Israel when they reported electrocardiographic indications of transient heart damage recorded during everyday activities such as sleeping and driving.

With the use of more reliable Holter techniques, the skepticism lessened. The Holter system was finally accepted by most cardiologists as a valid method for documenting ischemia when the reports of Drs. John Deanfield, Andrew Selwyn, and their colleagues from Dr. Attilio Maseri's research team at Hammersmith Hospital in London were published in 1983. What made these reports different from previous reports was that independent studies that used certain radioactive substances (radioisotopes) showed impaired blood flow to regions of the heart *at the same time* as the electrocardiographic abnormalities were taking place.

Armed with this type of confirmatory data, Drs. Deanfield, Selwyn and Maseri were able to demonstrate—as Drs. Schang and Pepine had done five years before—that for every episode of painful ischemia there were an average of four silent episodes. Based on these studies and those of other physician–scientists, it appears that anywhere from 25 to 100% of patients with painful angina have frequent episodes of silent ischemia. Taking 50% as an average figure, an estimated two million of the nation's four million angina patients have such episodes.

This is an impressive figure, one that dramatically challenges the way physicians treat patients. Should they treat the symptom of chest pain or should they treat the *total* number of *ischemic* episodes, regardless of whether pain is present? Take the case of Mr. Black, for example, typical of this type of patient. Originally diagnosed as having angina because of the oppressive chest pain that he experienced whenever he did heavy lifting on his construction job, Mr. Black was given standard heart medicines by his doctor. Soon after, he reported that the painful episodes seemed to have diminished markedly. At this point, the doctor felt he had treated the patient successfully, and, by traditional standards, he had. But when he read reports about silent ischemia in the medical journals, Mr. Black's doctor had second thoughts and he ordered a Holter monitor study. Over the course of 48 hours, he was surprised to find that Mr. Black had seven episodes of ischemia, each lasting from 2 to 12 minutes.

But Mr. Black was only aware of one of these episodes, according to the special diary he kept of his daily activities. His doctor realized the patient was not being adequately treated and changed his dosage of heart medicines accordingly.

So much for transient episodes of heart damage. What about the more lasting kind, the silent heart attack that we described in Mr. Brown's case in Chapter 1? There are a number of studies showing that at least 25% of the more than one million yearly heart attacks in the United States are unrecognized at the time they occur. The most well known of these reports is from the Framingham Study.

The town of Framingham, Massachusetts, was selected by the federally run Public Health Service in 1948 for a pioneering survey to determine the relation between the presence of "coronary risk factors" and future cardiac events. Five thousand of the town's residents formed the study group. At the time of entry into the study, none had evidence of heart disease. For the next four decades, these people underwent periodic examinations and answered questionnaires dealing with their social habits. For example, did they smoke? If so, how many cigarettes per day? The research showed that the frequency of future cardiac events such as death, heart attacks and development of angina could be statistically related to high blood pressure, cigarette smoking, high cholesterol levels in the blood and diabetes. Other factors such as obesity were also implicated but in a less statistically significant way.

The Framingham Study—and other similar epidemiologic studies done in other communities in the United States as well as foreign countries—helped establish the concept of coronary risk factors (see Chapter 3). An offshoot of the study was the surprising statistic that a good portion of the study population was showing up for their annual examinations without cardiac complaints but with unequivocal evidence of new heart attacks on the electrocardiogram! Despite careful questioning, the people involved could usually give no history suggestive of such an attack, although some did admit to vague malaise. Excluding the latter individuals, it was apparent that about one-quarter of the heart attacks that occurred in the Framingham Study population were silent, or, as they were termed, "unrecognized." Percentages from others studies ranged from 30 to 50%. It is not clear from these reports exactly how many people have had an unrecognized heart attack as their only manifestation of coronary artery disease, but with over one million heart attacks occurring yearly in the United States, it is obvious that the figure is at least in the hundreds of thousands. Some of these persons will go on to other cardiac events occurring at about the same rate as people with symptomatic heart attacks. Hence, this type of heart attack—assuming the patient survives the initial event—is far from benign.

——— 3 ———

Detection of Painful and Silent Heart Disease: Risk Factors and Diagnostic Procedures

The most important clues to the early detection of heart disease include cigarette smoking, high blood levels of cholesterol, high blood pressure, diabetes and a family history of "premature" heart attacks (before the age of 55 or 60). In individuals with one or more of these risk factors, an electrocardiogram recorded during exertion (the exercise or stress test) can be a valuable screening procedure to detect silent heart disease, especially when confirmed with radioisotopic procedures. The coronary arteriogram is still the procedure of choice, however, for the most precise anatomic localization of coronary artery blockages in both painful and silent heart disease.

———————

Most visitors to the city of Pisa in northern Italy have one thought in mind: They want to see the famed Leaning Tower. To be sure, there are other tourist attractions in the city and its environs, but they are usually secondary considerations. But when cardiologists from around the world came to Pisa in the

1970s, seeing the Leaning Tower was not their primary motive; they were there to visit the clinical and research facilities of the University of Pisa's medical school. There, under the leadership of Dr. Attilio Maseri, a team of cardiologists were involved in some of the most important investigations of coronary artery disease ever performed in this century.

Dr. Maseri and his group were studying the phenomenon of *coronary vasospasm*—sudden, total obstruction of human coronary arteries due to intense constriction of the muscle cells in the walls of the arteries. They were studying this phenomenon both in the relatively small number of patients who have it in its purest form in which it occurs only in the resting state (this is termed "Prinzmetal's angina" after the Los Angeles cardiologist who discovered it), as well as in the much more numerous patients with common exertion-related angina. The uniqueness of their studies resulted from their comprehensive use of very sophisticated techniques to monitor their patients' cardiac function.

What they found in their patients was to have profound effects on the very basis of our concept that ischemia was always painful. They found that frequent, and often severe, derangements of cardiac function were occurring in their patients and, as expected, were invariably accompanied by electrocardiographic changes—but not by pain! Pain was infrequent; generally, these were silent ischemic episodes. It was largely as a result of these landmark studies that continuous electrocardiographic monitoring of patients with coronary artery disease was begun at several research centers. When Dr. Maseri moved to the Hammersmith Hospital in London in 1979 to become the Sir John McMichael Professor in Cardiovascular Medicine at the Royal Postgraduate Medical School, he continued his studies of silent ischemia with his associate from Pisa, Dr. Sergio Chierchia,* as well as British investigators like Dr. John Deanfield. When we

---

*By 1992, both investigators had returned to Italy to head cardiology centers in Rome (Maseri) and Milan (Chierchia).

met Dr. Maseri in London, we asked him what his thoughts were that day in 1972 when he first witnessed an episode of silent ischemia.

"I remember seeing an abnormality that I usually associate with pain on the electrocardiographic monitor at the nurse's station outside the patient's room. I rushed inside to find him calmly reading a book. 'Do you have pain?' I asked. 'Who me?' he said, obviously very surprised. 'No, no pain.' I went back to the monitor and the huge injury wave was still there. A nitroglycerin under the tongue made it go away just as it would if he had pain. That convinced me it was really ischemia. Later we found a whole series of these events in patients and proved they were ischemia with radioisotopic studies. In 1977, we started using Holter monitors, and we've even observed silent infarctions in our patients! Why they have no pain, I don't know. Sometimes the painless episodes are short and not too severe, but other times they're very long. Something must be interfering with the transmission of the pain impulse."

Holter studies are just one of the electrocardiographic ways of detecting silent ischemia. Before an electrocardiogram is performed, the physician usually interviews the patient. Physicians are not supermen or superwomen. Just as they cannot wave a magic wand over an ill patient and announce that the patient is cured, they also cannot look at—and talk to—an apparently healthy person and decide whether or not that person does or does not have silent heart disease. No amount of questioning, and virtually nothing found on physical examination, can be automatically linked to underlying heart disease in most asymptomatic persons who have such a condition. How then can the physician make the diagnosis?

One of the clues is whether or not there is a family history of "premature" coronary artery disease. Premature refers to the development of angina or a heart attack—or a fatal cardiac arrhythmia (irregularity of the heartbeat)—before the age at which these events usually occur (i.e., 60–65 years of age or older). These events are not "normal" in the older age group—cardiologists never consider heart disease a normal situation—but we know they are associated with the aging process.

The changes that occur in the blood vessels of the body with time, the thickening of the vessel walls and the narrowing of the internal channel through which the blood passes, are a result of a combination of factors (see Chapter 4). When these changes are accelerated in persons between the ages of 35 and 55 (or 35–60 as some physicians prefer) we call the resulting heart disease "premature."

Physicians do not expect to deal with these conditions in such relatively young people. Therefore, when an apparently healthy person is talking to a physician about family history, and in reply to questions about the health of grandparents, parents, uncles and aunts, rather matter-of-factly notes that his father's brother, Uncle John, had a heart attack at age 52 and that his father's other brother, Uncle Sid, died without apparent cause at age 48, a physician's ears will perk up.

"How old was your grandfather when he died?" he will ask.

"Seventy-two."

"And what did he die of?"

"A stroke; my father had one five years ago at 65, but my father's still alive."

Strokes are due to obstructive disease in the arteries leading to the brain or those in the brain itself. They are "first cousins" to heart attacks. This patient has painted a picture of cardiovascular disease in the family. (Usually it is "his" family rather than "hers." Heart disease in women is very uncommon before the age of 55, unless there is an inherited problem with breakdown of body cholesterol by the liver. In that situation, the blood cholesterol levels are often very high in childhood and in the teenage years, and heart attacks are common in the early and mid-adult years.)

The finding of a history of cardiovascular disease in the family, especially in middle-aged rather than only elderly relatives, should be a red flag to the physician, a warning that the apparently "normal" person in the opposite chair may already be a silent victim of the same process and soon may be a not-so-silent victim!

The public as a whole perceives of family history only in its most positive form: My parents lived into their 80s; therefore, I probably will also. If one or both of the parents died of heart disease at an early age, the person is likely to dismiss it as something that probably will not also befall him because of advances in medical or surgical treatment. This is a fallacious argument. For one thing, if one's parents did indeed live into their 80s free of heart disease, there is no guarantee that their 40-year-old son, who unlike them smokes like the proverbial chimney and loves his beefsteaks heavily marbled with fat, will follow in their long-lived footsteps. Furthermore, the individual with the short-lived parents may not be able to count on advances in medical care unless his silent disease can be detected before it kills or cripples him. He must learn about the value of screening procedures and he must learn about—and adopt— healthy living habits to retard or prevent the disease process.

The education of the public in these matters is the responsibility of the physician, but often the physician falls woefully short of expectations. Preventing disease simply doesn't interest most doctors as much as treating disease. They feel it is not their "problem;" it's for the public health professionals—those guys in preventive medicine—to worry about.

In addition to a family history of premature heart disease, the other warning signal that can be found on a routine checkup is the presence of one or more of the coronary risk factors. High blood pressure (hypertension), cigarette smoking, diabetes and high cholesterol levels in the blood were defined as the primary risk factors by large-scale epidemiologic surveys; that is, follow-up studies of selected populations in which these and other factors could be correlated with the subsequent development of cardiac events (angina, heart attacks or death due to heart disease).

At the time of the Framingham Study, knowledge of coronary risk factors was very circumstantial. "Clustering" of certain factors had been found in people who had already had heart attacks. This suggested that there might be an association between these factors and the development of heart disease, but proof was lacking. For this reason, in 1948 the United States government chose the Public Health Service to conduct an on-going population study in a representative American community (Framingham, Massachusetts). All enrollees in the study would have pertinent family history, personal characteristics and health habits recorded and evaluated. As we noted in Chapter 2 when we discussed silent heart attacks, there were 5000 subjects in the original study. At that time, the town's entire population was just under 36,000, so the enrollees represented a good chunk of the citizenry. They also represented a cross section of occupations.

Because Framingham is only about 20 miles away from Boston, one of the major centers for medical research, the United States Public Health Service was able to enlist the support of faculty from two of Boston's three medical schools (Boston University Medical School and Harvard Medical School) in the study. When the National Institutes of Health was formed by the government several years later, they also participated with the Public Health Service and those medical schools in evaluating the data.

It soon became apparent that several important trends were emerging. People who developed cardiovascular disease (heart disease or strokes) in Framingham were more likely to be cigarette smokers; have high blood pressure, high blood cholesterol and diabetes; be obese and physically inactive. Sorting out the more important of these factors required what is known as multivariate risk analysis, a mathematical technique useful in "weeding out" the less important factors.

In the final analysis, several elements had to be present before it was valid to call something a "coronary risk factor." The risk factor had to be present before there were any signs of the disease (painful or silent), and the risk had to increase with longer exposure to the factor. If reversal of the factor led to a decrease in the incidence of the disease, it would be considered additional validating evidence, as would data linking the factor to the experimental production of coronary heart disease in animals. Finally, whatever was observed in Framingham would have to be confirmed in other populations in different areas of the United States and abroad. Only when all these criteria were fulfilled could one be confident in labelling a factor a likely contributor to heart disease.

What came out of the Framingham Study was that not only could the major risk factors be shown to be associated with the development of cardiac events *independent* of the presence of other risk factors (this was learned through use of multivariate analysis), but the risk factors also acted *synergistically*; that is, the combination of two or more was worse than any one alone. A coronary risk profile was worked out to enable individuals to plot their own relative risk; it was published as the *Coronary Risk Handbook* by the American Heart Association. For example, if an individual has a blood pressure reading slightly above the normal range but doesn't smoke or have an elevated blood cholesterol level, he or she has twice the risk of developing a heart attack as someone with a normal blood pressure reading. A one pack-a-day cigarette smoker with normal blood pressure and normal blood cholesterol also has twice the risk of a non-smoker. Someone with a cholesterol level just above "average" ("average" is not necessarily normal, as we will discuss in Chapter 7) also has twice the risk of someone who has a level well below the average value for that age group. Put all three risk factors together and the risk increases from twofold to tenfold!

What makes these statistics so depressing is that high blood pressure, high cholesterol levels and cigarette smoking are all correctable—as is one of the minor but still important risk factors, obesity. Obesity is not only related to overeating, but also to physical inactivity, two disappointingly common features of American society. Foreign visitors often voice amazement at the number of massively obese people under 40 in our country (ever been to Disneyland?). Obesity also contributes to the development of high blood pressure and heart disease. Even people who may be genetically overweight can reduce their food intake to cut down on the risk of heart disease.

The other important minor risk factors are increasing age and male sex. Obviously, these are not "correctable." As we noted in Chapter 2, pre-menopausal women have a much lower incidence of heart disease than do men of a similar age. This advantage can be offset, however, by improper attention to good health habits. In particular, the combination of cigarette smoking and birth-control pills (both of which can lead to enhanced blood clotting) increases a young woman's risk for cardiovascular disease at a time in her life when this is normally not a problem. Once a woman loses the protective effect of the pre-menopausal years, then the cumulative effect of cigarette smoking and the other risk factors begin to take their toll—but again, most are correctable (see Chapter 13 for more details).

Are the risk factor data confined to the United States? No. For example, the Seven Countries Study was conducted by Dr. Ancel Keys in the 1960s to examine the importance of cholesterol in the blood. This study established that differences in coronary artery disease between one country and another could be related to differences in diets and blood cholesterol levels. Smaller studies in other cities, and other countries, have also confirmed this association. The importance of risk factors in detecting coronary artery disease—or at least suggesting the possibility that coronary artery disease will develop—brings us back to a consideration of family history as a risk factor.

Any systematic attempt to evaluate the role of family history involves certain problems. First, patients and their relatives have to supply their own diagnosis. How can we be sure that Aunt Jane really did die of a heart attack? Without a death certificate—or even more precise autopsy data—we can't. The other major problem is how to decide whether heart disease in a given family is due to some confounding environmental variable such as cigarette smoking rather than to inherited tendencies.

Once heart disease has been identified in a family, can we be sure that it is really an independent variable and not totally dependent on an inherited predisposition to hypertension or high blood cholesterol? In a 1984 study, Dr. Steven Shea and his colleagues at Presbyterian Hospital in New York City devised a protocol to test the hypothesis that family history is an independent risk factor, especially in persons who would otherwise be considered at low risk. Over 200 patients who had documented coronary artery disease on coronary arteriograms were questioned about heart disease or sudden death in natural parents or siblings. Their responses were contrasted to those of 57 control subjects who had no coronary artery disease on cardiac catheterization. These 57 patients had undergone coronary arteriography during evaluation for other kinds of heart disease, such as valvular heart disease. Both the coronary and the control subjects were assigned risk scores based on their blood pressure, level of cholesterol and other standard risk factors. As expected, the control subjects had lower risk scores than the coronary subjects; also as expected, the relatives of the coronary patients had higher risk scores than the relatives of the controls. To minimize the confounding effect of the standard risk factors, a comparison was then made between coronary subjects and control subjects with the *same* risk score grouping. The new finding was that relatives of coronary subjects in the 50–65 age group had a four-to sixfold greater probability of having a heart attack than relatives of control subjects in the 50–65 age group and this was despite very similar risk scores.

Other than learning about the patient's family history and presence of coronary risk factors from measuring blood pressure and blood cholesterol levels, are there any other ways that physicians can detect heart disease in persons who otherwise appear to be healthy? Unfortunately, there are few telltale signs on physical examination. One of these signs, however, is a dead give-away. On the skin in the corner of the eye, near the nose, one can observe whitish yellow raised patches the size of a pea in some persons with elevated cholesterol levels. Not all persons with elevated cholesterol levels have these patches, but when present, they are remarkably accurate predictors of cholesterol levels in the range that will sooner or later usually result in coronary artery disease. The other major finding is related to blood pressure. When there are signs of damage to the heart, brain, blood vessels and kidneys, the physician knows that high blood pressure has been present for long periods of time— although in most instances, the affected persons are not aware of high blood pressure. It begins and progresses insiduously, a truly silent disease for much of its course.

Measuring blood pressure, finding signs of high cholesterol (and confirming it with the appropriate blood tests), noting a history of cigarette smoking—all of these provide evidence that a person is at risk for heart disease. But they do not provide proof that the disease is already present, although silent. Unless the patient has a clear-cut history of intermittent bouts of typical chest pain or has suffered a heart attack, there is still no proof of active disease. However, evidence of prior damage—even when silent—can be obtained with the electrocardiogram (often abbreviated ECG, or EKG from the German).

Electrocardiograms in one form or another—the conventional "resting" tracing, the 24-hour or longer ambulatory (Holter) monitor, the exercise (stress) tracing—are so important—in fact, so vital—to the appreciation of coronary artery disease in humans that some knowledge of the history of this remarkable device is helpful.

The mechanism that initiates a heart muscle beat (contraction) involves transmission of a small amount of electric current generated within the heart. This is an inherent feature not only of the heart as a whole, but also of its component tissue cells. Remove the heart from the body and it will continue to beat; cut the isolated heart into small pieces and they will continue to beat. There is one area that beats faster than others in the normal heart. This is the *cardiac pacemaker*, a small, almost microscopic collection of special cells located in the right atrium, one of the two collecting chambers for blood in the heart. From this pacemaker, a wave of electrical excitation (current) travels in an orderly manner through the rest of the heart and particularly through the left ventricle (the main pumping chamber) via a system of specialized conducting tracts or bundles. Impulses can travel as fast as

4000 mm/sec in some of the specified cells that make up these bundles. (The artificial electric pacemaker required by some patients is really a poor imitation of the heart's own pacemaker.)

The electrocardiogram is simply a graphic representation of the heart's electrical activity. The electrical forces of the heart often, but not always, provide data as to its function and anatomic state. Thus, the electrocardiogram is an *indirect* measure of heart function. To record the electrical activity at different sites, metallic electrodes are attached to the arms, legs and chest of the patient. The electrodes and their connecting cables (plus a central terminal) carry the electrical forces of the heart (not the arms and legs) from the skin to the recording machine. Because the electrodes not only record electrical activity from the part of the heart closest to the electrode but from *all* the electrical forces of the heart at a given instant, this electrical field is in reality a balance of forces (called vectors) consisting of augmenting and opposing forces.

Fortunately for physicians and patients, the early developers of the electrocardiogram, William Einthoven of the Netherlands, Sir Thomas Lewis of Great Britain and Frank Wilson of the United States, were able to correlate the electrocardiographic wave forms with contractions of various parts of the heart. This led to its first great clinical use, the determination of normal and abnormal heart rhythms—which is really the sequence of conduction from the pacemaker to other regions of the heart. Later in the twentieth century, other investigators were able to identify cardiac diseases (such as heart attacks) by the electrocardiographic "patterns" that the full 12-lead tracing documented.

For our purposes, the key findings lie in the lines on the tracing called the QRS complex (ventricular contraction) and the ST segment (ventricular relaxation). When a portion of the heart dies, the QRS complex becomes abnormal; when the heart muscle is temporarily injured—enough to cause an alteration in current flow—the ST segment becomes abnormal (an injury current). Unfortunately, there are also other cardiac and noncardiac causes of QRS and ST abnormalities, so the cardiologist's job is not quite as simple as it may appear!

As great a tool as the electrocardiogram is, it must never be forgotten that it does have its limitations as a recording device, and that *unless the electrocardiogram is recorded during some type of exertion, it has little value as a screening procedure for detecting latent (silent) heart disease.* Too many physicians will perform a resting electrocardiogram as part of their examination of the patient, see that it is normal and pronounce the patient fit. Nothing could be more misleading! Unless the electrocardiogram is recorded during a patient's daily activities (or a standard exercise test), having a normal tracing conveys nothing about blockages in the coronary circulation. It requires only a moment's reflection to realize the absurdity of using the standard electrocardiogram to detect heart disease. The patient is lying comfortably at rest on an examining table during the test. In this setting, the test is useless (unless there has been prior damage to the heart, which can then be detected on the resting electrocardiogram). Often in a patient with known heart disease, the resting electrocardiogram records changes that may have occurred in the interim between visits. This can be helpful, and we certainly have no quarrel with its use in this setting. But in an apparently healthy person, unless we detect an unrecognized heart attack, we have learned nothing. What might we be missing? There may be an obstruction in a blood vessel that is so severe that a heart attack may be imminent, yet a normal, resting electrocardiogram will present no clues to this possibility.

It is for this reason that the exercise test has become such an important component of the workup of an asymptomatic person suspected of having heart disease. The key word here is suspected, for the exercise test—like nearly all of the specialized tests of medical sciences—is not perfect. There are false-positive results (the test is abnormal but no coronary artery disease can be found) and false-negative results (the test is normal but coronary artery disease is present). To use the exercise test for its maximal value, the physician has to know for what it is being used (not as silly as it sounds) and then select the appropriate testing group. For example, in a patient with a history of heart attacks and angina, the test would not be used to diagnose coronary artery disease, since the physician already knows it to be present, but rather to assess its severity (in a way that we will discuss shortly). On the other hand, when a physician is considering the diagnosis of coronary artery disease in an apparently healthy individual, the index of suspicion for believing silent coronary artery disease is present must be high. This means that *one or more coronary risk factors should be present and/or*, as we have discussed, *there is a family history of coronary artery disease*, preferably of the premature type. Age and sex must also be taken into consideration since coronary disease is more common in men and increases with age. It is very rare in most women under 35, and under age 60 still much more common in men. Women also present special problems in relation to interpretation of the test: false-positive results are more numerous. The reasons for this are unknown.

The rationale for careful selection of patients to be tested is based on Bayes's theorem (from the eighteenth century English philosopher Thomas Bayes). This theorem states that the predictive value of a positive (abnormal) test is influenced not only by the sensitivity of the test but also the prevalence of the disease to be tested for in the population under study. If the probability of having the disease—even before the test is administered—is very high (for example, a group of patients with prior heart attacks would have over a 90% likelihood of having coronary artery disease) then so too will the post-test probability that an abnormal test reflects heart disease. In other words, the likelihood of having disease would go from 90% to 97%. If, however, there is only a 5% prevalence of disease (as in an asymptomatic population) a positive test might only change that to 20%, as confirmed by coronary arteriograms. For these reasons, we not only preselect the asymptomatic patients most likely to have disease (based on risk factors), but we also interpret the test in a graded fashion, rather than in a "postive-negative" or "disease/no disease" manner. Some of the things we look for are severity of the ST segment abnormality, its appearance early in the test and its persistence into the recovery period. This increases the likelihood from 20% to closer to 80%, which is a more reasonable figure on which to make a diagnosis.

The exercise test itself is now quite standardized with guidelines including how long the test should last. Although a treadmill is now the most popular method of testing, this was not always the case. The first device was the Masters two-step, introduced by Dr. Arthur Masters over 40 years ago. Individuals walked at a brisk pace up and down two wooden steps with electrodes attached to arms and legs. The number of trips was determined by age. The "recovery" period after the test began by having the patient lie down, with the chest leads attached immediately upon stopping exercise.

An upright, stationary bicycle, with a device to control pedal resistance, was the next method used. Here the patient cycles against a slowly increasing resistance. This is still employed in many hospitals because it is cheaper, requires less space and is quieter than the treadmill.

The treadmill is the newest and most popular innovation. A variety of protocols for increasing the speed and incline of the treadmill have been tested in the last 15 years. They are named after the physicians who devised them. The Bruce protocol is the most widely used, followed by the modified Bruce and the Naughton protocols. These are for patients not capable of full activity, for example, after a heart attack or heart surgery. In all protocols, patients exercise until either symptoms or fatigue set in (this is called a maximal test) or to a set heart rate that depends on their age (sub-maximal test). Prior to the test, the patient is instructed in how the treadmill works, asked to wear soft shoes and cautioned not to eat for several hours before the test. This is primarily to avoid nausea and vomiting that sometimes accompanies myocardial ischemia. The electrocardiographic findings during the test are displayed on a computer screen located near the treadmill. The patient's heart rate is also displayed on the screen. Blood pressure measurements are taken at regular intervals both to add an extra measure of safety and also to correlate with the electrocardiographic results. Despite the fact that ischemia occurs in many tests, the exercise test is a remarkably safe procedure. Only rarely does a heart attack result and fatalities occur in only about one in 10,000 tests.

In research studies, the results of the exercise test have often been compared with coronary arteriograms, the "gold standard" for diagnosing coronary artery disease. The first large-scale study to compare exercise test results with the coronary arteriographic findings in the same patients was performed by a group of investigators led by one of the authors (PFC) at the Peter Bent Brigham Hospital in Boston. Over 300 patients were described in a report published in 1972. This was not only the largest series reported to that time, but it was also the last to use the two-step device.

Our study was motivated by some interesting data from the life-insurance industry. Their statistics had shown that individuals who had had an abnormal (positive) exercise test tended to have shorter life spans—a finding of obvious importance to the life insurance companies, since the results can be used to calculate actuarial tables that determine premium fees. The reason for the results was not clear, but these observations (that a positive exercise test was *not* a good marker for longevity) were to be repeated over and over in subsequent years. Whenever healthy populations were subjected to exercise testing, those with abnormal responses had a greater chance of dying over the course of the follow-up period than did those with normal responses.

Our goal in 1972 was to use a large enough sample to confirm results of previously reported small-scale studies that had correlated exercise tests with coronary arteriograms. We hoped to end speculation about the meaning of abnormal responses in patients with chest pain complaints, and the results did indeed confirm earlier findings in a very dramatic way! Of 49 patients with the most marked abnormality on the exercise test, all 49 had coronary artery disease on the arteriogram and 35 (70%) had the most severe form of blockages—the most extensive and the most life-threatening. With lesser degrees of abnormalities on the exercise test, we found fewer instances of severe coronary artery disease and more instances of milder disease, and even some "normal" subjects (people with chest pain complaints but no blockages in their coronary arteries). With a negative exercise test, we found mostly normal subjects or those with mild disease. The results showed that the reason that people with very positive tests faired poorly in the life-insurance studies was because they had the most disease. It was as simple as that.

A problem with the 1972 study—and, for that matter, all studies that used the two-step device—was that a good number of the patients evaluated (about 20%) had neither positive nor negative results but rather something in between. Usually this meant that they completed the required number of steps without either developing specific abnormalities on the electrocardiogram (called ST segment depression) or achieving the necessary target heart rate that made the test truly negative. Use of the bicycle, and later the treadmill, helped overcome this problem of inadequate stress to the patient's cardiovascular system.

We also looked at additional measurements besides ST segment depression. Again, our interest was piqued by reports that the length of time over which the abnormalities persisted, as well as the time at which they occurred, was an important marker of blocked coronary arteries. Later in the 1970s, our center combined a series of these measurements into indexes and applied them to the results of treadmill testing. It was then possible to show that lesser degrees of ST segment depression could also mean extensive coronary artery disease if, for example, they occurred within the first six minutes of the exercise test and/or lasted at least six minutes into the recovery period. These studies have subsequently been confirmed at many other centers.

The attempt to obtain a diagnostic index based on exercise test results was not new; in fact, we had constructed one in 1972 combining the exercise test results with the cholesterol level and the results of other easily obtained clinical tests. But, of course, all this work had been done in patients complaining of chest pain, though some were atypical for heart disease. The rapidly emerging challenge was to apply these lessons to the asymptomatic population. Here, because of Bayes's theorem of probability, cardiologists knew they would be on softer ground. More "hard" data confirming the ischemic nature of the ECG findings were needed. This data would have to be obtained whenever possible without subjecting asymptomatic patients to coronary arteriography solely on the basis of ST segment changes.

The techniques that were developed in the late 1960s and that became widespread in the 1970s and 1980s involved the use of small amounts of radioactive substances (such as thallium-201) called isotopes. By injecting solutions of these substances mixed with saline (salt water) into the bloodstream, it was possible to visualize their appearance in the heart by means of special X-ray-like cameras. These *gamma cameras* measure the emission of radioactive gamma particles. With some techniques, the radioactive substance was found in the heart muscle—if its blood supply was normal. Thallium-201 is chemically similar to substances that are normally present in both the blood and the heart muscle. Because of their similar chemical makeup, the heart tissue cannot distinguish one substance from the other and allows both substances to pass freely through the cell membrane that regulates to-and-fro passage of chemicals and other biological materials. If blood supply is abnormal, however, as it is in coronary artery disease, then thallium-201 will not be present in the affected region. A "hole" or blank space will be present on the special X-ray picture of the heart. This blank space will correspond to the area where the coronary artery is partially or totally blocked.

One of the fascinating aspects of this technique is that the blank spaces can be transient in their appearance, just as the electrocardiographic abnormalities are. For example, if a person exercises, and the resulting thallium X-rays show a blank space, it is not at all unusual to take another X-ray two hours later and find no blank space at all! Once the ischemia has passed, the remaining thallium can enter the heart uniformly since blood flow is normal.

Probably no one in the United States has done more work in the area of thallium imaging than Dr. George Beller, now at the

University of Virginia. In the course of his studies with this technique in patients who have angina or who are recovering from heart attacks or heart surgery, he has also looked at the problem of how to verify exercise ST segment abnormalities in asymptomatic persons without necessarily subjecting them to coronary arteriography. One of the ways to do this is to repeat the exercise test, administer thallium at the height of exercise, take the special X-ray immediately and repeat the X-ray again several hours later. In one such study, performed with colleagues at Massachusetts General Hospital in 1981, 35 men and women between the ages of 35 and 60, who had positive but painless standard exercise tests, were retested with the thallium technique. Twenty-four (15 women and 9 men) had no defects (blank spaces) in their thallium images. When those 24 patients were subsequently subjected to coronary arteriography to confirm the validity of the thallium results, 23 had no appreciable coronary atherosclerosis. The remaining patient had one partial obstruction in a non-major vessel.

The 11 patients (8 men and 3 women) with thallium defects had a far different arteriographic profile. Eight clearly had critical blockages in one or more coronary arteries, and two others had lesser degrees of disease. Only one (a woman) had no disease. The reason for the false-positive thallium test in the women was a condition called mitral valve prolapse, a fluttering of one of the heart valves that is quite common in women but is only rarely of clinical importance even in those persons who have chest pain because of it.

Another of Dr. Beller's goals was to see if these "non-invasive" test procedures were more cost-effective than the very reliable but expensive "invasive" procedure, cardiac catheterization (which includes the coronary arteriography described in Chapter 1). As Dr. Beller explained:

"I was very surprised at first to learn that abnormal thallium scans in a group of asymptomatic persons with positive electrocardiographic findings were reliable indicators of serious disease on the coronary arteriogram. I clearly remember one self-referred man, age 50, with coronary risk factors. He turned out to have disease of all three major coronary arteries. As time went by, we saw many more like him. I wasn't surprised any more!"

"What about studies in post-heart attack patients?" we asked.

"This is where the thallium scan is also very helpful. Regardless of pain during the test, regardless of electrocardiographic changes, abnormal thallium scans are by themselves extremely reliable predictors of future cardiac events. This is probably because the test is often abnormal at very low levels of activities, which is the activity level patients follow out-of-hospital, and because the perfusion abnormalities occur before electrocardiographic changes or pain."

The reader may wonder why physicians bother with a standard test at all if the thallium-stress test is so reliable. The answer is some don't bother with it! They use the thallium stress test as their initial screening procedure when a stress test is indicated. But because the thallium stress test is more expensive and requires more sophisticated recording and interpreting equipment, many physicians prefer the standard exercise test as the initial test. In addition, it is often possible to perform the standard stress test in a physician's office or clinic and obtain immediate results. The thallium stress test usually requires a more specialized setting. Furthermore, we haven't yet achieved 100% accuracy with this test, despite its impressive results. As Dr. Beller concluded, "The ultimate test is one that is inexpensive and specific. When it's negative, we can rest assured that coronary disease is not present."

The other non-invasive procedure using radioisotopes is called the radionuclide ventriculogram, or RVG for short. *Radionuclide* is another term for radioisotope, and *ventriculogram* refers to an X-ray picture, or nuclear image, of the left or right ventricle (the pumping chambers of the heart). Just like thallium, the radioisotope for this procedure (technetium pertechnetate) is injected into a vein, but, unlike thallium, it is an inert substance. It stays within the bloodstream instead of diffusing into heart muscle cells. As a result, the image obtained is one of the cavities of the ventricles. One can "see" the pumping chambers expand as blood enters from the reservoir chambers (the atria) and then contract when the heart muscle propels the blood from the heart out to peripheral organs. If the recording computer flashes the expansion–contraction images quickly, a movie-like effect is obtained. The heart appears to be beating. Abnormalities in how it beats can then be analyzed visually or by the computer.

There are a variety of techniques by which this analysis can be done, but the important point for the patient is that it does not involve the insertion of catheters into the heart. An example of how this technique is useful in persons free of heart symptoms was reported in 1983 by our research group at the State University of New York Health Sciences Center at Stony Brook. In that study, we compared wall motion abnormalities in a group of patients with and without symptoms, all of whom had severe blockages in their coronary arteries. The wall motion abnormalities were brought on by exercise using a specific protocol with a bicycle, and the radioisotope images were obtained before and immediately after the exercise. We found the same degree of abnormality in both groups of patients. In other words, it didn't matter whether pain was produced during the exercise test. Other investigators have reported similar findings. Like the thallium test, the RVG can localize the area of impaired blood supply: The abnormal wall motion will correspond to that part of the ventricle supplied by a partially or totally blocked coronary artery. Like the thallium test, this is an expensive procedure. Hence, it is not done as a first step, but rather as a way of obtaining more pertinent data in a person already being evaluated. One of the more exciting recent developments has been the introduction of a *portable* RVG that is worn in a vest-like apparatus—termed the VEST—and can record wall motion changes during daily life just like the Holter monitor can record ECG changes.

The radioisotope procedures complement the exercise electrocardiogram and usually verify its findings. Once non-invasive testing is completed, a decision may be made to proceed to coronary arteriography—an invasive procedure with some risk.

Sometimes, however, the Holter monitor can be helpful in this situation. As we noted in Chapter 2, it served for many years primarily as a way to study heart rhythm abnormalities. Patients who complained of dizziness or fainting spells or "skipped beats" in their pulse might have totally normal electrocardiograms taken in the conventional manner. The Holter monitor can record 24 hours at a time, with the taped data being stored on a small reel of tape and then played back rapidly through a scanning device.

Only in the last 10 years have attempts been made to study ST segment abnormalities during daily life, as well as rhythm disturbances. In a sense, this is ironic, since the first scientific paper about this device illustrated transient abnormalities (ST segment depression) rather than rhythm disturbances! These electrocardiographic changes, so vividly described by Dr. Maseri earlier in the chapter, had first been observed on bedside monitors. Chapter 2 introduced the reader to some of the early studies in which the Holter monitor was used to evaluate coronary artery disease. Foremost among these were the 1974 and 1975 studies from Drs. Dan Tzivoni and Shlomo Stern, then at Hadassah Hospital in Jerusalem. Those two physicians had the ingenious idea of monitoring the daily activities of their coronary patients with this device. They were amazed to learn that throughout the course of the day, myocardial ischemia was not a rarity—as one would think from the relatively few attacks of chest pain that their patients had—but rather commonplace. Most of the time, however, no pain accompanied the ischemia. We recently asked Dr. Stern about those earlier studies.

"Driving a car in the city was a part of our patients' everyday activities, a very stressful part of modern living. We were not at all surprised that it aggravated their heart disease, but, of course, we didn't expect such a low incidence of painful episodes compared to the silent ones."

In Chapter 2, we alluded to the fact that their results did not meet with widespread acceptance. Criticisms were mainly technical in nature and questioned the reliability of the Holter device in recording ST segment abnormalities, which are very prone to change when body position changes, a person coughs, and so on. At the time, Dr. Stern felt that such criticism was justified. Today, with the development of more reliable equipment, these objections have been largely overcome. He is now interested in applying this technique to the high-risk, asymptomatic person.

Another reason the Holter device now enjoys increasing use both in research and as a clinical tool is because of the Hammersmith Hospital studies cited in Chapter 2. We asked Dr. Deanfield how he became interested in Holter monitoring.

"Most of a patient's activities occur out of the hospital. It only seemed logical to look for ST depression during that time, as well as when the patient is in the hospital. To have an impact on mortality in coronary artery disease, to avoid damage to the heart and death, we should not simply wait for symptoms to occur. We must find out if ischemia detected on a daily basis matters to the patient in terms of prognosis. How should he alter his life, what treatment should he take?"

"What about the future?" we asked.

"Because we are obligated now to detect ischemia and to look for it aggressively, we need a new generation of real-time Holter-type devices that are more 'physician-friendly' and more 'patient-friendly' than the current models."

In fact, these newer devices are now available with microprocessors using computer chips. They can provide on-line ("real-time") summaries of electrocardiographic abnormalities as they occur, thus doing away with cumbersome reel analysis.

As the reader probably has predicted by this time, not only are patients with chest pain being assessed for the frequency and duration of their silent episodes of heart damage, but persons without symptoms are now being studied as well. One such study was recently completed at Stony Brook. Because of our interest in silent heart disease, the center has become a referral center for this syndrome. Persons from surrounding communities who have been identified by their family doctors, internists or cardiologists as having this problem are studied by us. They participate in one of the research protocols designed to learn as much as possible about this disorder. The first 10 asymptomatic patients to complete our special Holter research protocol formed the basis for our 1987 report. Prior to the Holter part of the protocol, they underwent stress testing (with positive, but silent, abnormalities) and coronary arteriography (demonstrating significant disease in one or more of their major coronary arteries). Three of the patients had had prior heart attacks but were then asymptomatic; the other seven patients had never had any symptoms. These 10 patients were studied intensively with the Holter monitor, often wearing the device for several 48-hour periods.

What was observed on the Holter monitors was both surprising and alarming. These apparently well individuals were having anywhere from 1 to 17 episodes of myocardial ischemia per 48-hour monitoring period—all without symptoms! In other words, they were having a similar pattern of out-of-hospital transient heart damage that was similar to the patients with angina and silent ischemia reported by others several years earlier. Many episodes on Holter monitoring lasted for only several minutes in these asymptomatic persons, but others were longer, some up to a half-hour! Whether or not these transient—but long—episodes could result in heart attacks with severe heart damage was not clear from these initial studies, but, like so much else about silent heart disease, they are provocative in their implications. As Dr. Deanfield wondered, do these episodes influence prognosis? Should treatment be started immediately?

The answers to these questions remain unclear, but what the studies clearly demonstrate is the need for intensive study of silent heart disease in order to detect it as completely as possible. In our center, the patients undergo coronary arteriography when the non-invasive studies, including Holter monitoring, strongly point to the probability of having disease. We try to avoid catheterizing people who have only a small chance of having disease. This reluctance is related to the risks of coronary arteriography. Unlike the exercise test, the thallium stress test or the exercise radionuclide ventriculogram, which are only rarely associated with fatalities (1 in 10,000 procedures), the risks are higher with the coronary arteriogram. Patients planning to undergo any of these procedures should first discuss the risks with their physicians; this is especially true of the coronary arteriogram.

Before describing what the specific risks of the coronary arteriogram are, it would be useful to review the background of this procedure. This vital key to understanding how the heart works owes much to the courage of a young German physician, Werner Forssman. In 1929, he passed a catheter through a vein in his left arm and guided it by an X-ray camera until it entered his right atrium. He documented what he had done by walking a flight of stairs to the X-ray department and having a chest X-ray taken of himself! Instead of being praised for his action, he was criticized for doing something foolish and potentially dangerous. He repeated the experiment several times but eventually gave up his interest in it and completed his medical training as a urologist. His work stimulated others, however, and the era of cardiac catheterization began. It was not until the end of World War II that the next major breakthrough took place. Drs. Andre Cournard and Dickinson Richards, working in Bellevue Hospital in New York City, investigated pressure and flow in various heart chambers. For their contribution to understanding how the heart works, they (along with Forssman) received the Nobel Prize for medicine and physiology in 1956.

In 1959, the modern phase of cardiac catheterization was launched with injections of a chemical, called a dye or contrast agent that can be seen on X-rays, into the coronary arteries. The use of a contrast agent to visualize the coronary arteries and the various chambers of the heart is commonplace today. Because the dye replaces blood for several seconds (and for other reasons as well) the procedure has some risk attached to it. Today, given the development of improved technology and safer dyes, this risk is very small. It is generally accepted that in a properly equipped, adequately staffed and well-used cardiac catheterization laboratory, the risk of a serious complication (stroke, heart attack or death) is less than 1%. "Well-used" is an important consideration and means that there should be a certain number of cases done per year to insure continuing proficiency by the staff. New

York State law, for example, requires a minimum of 200 cases per year for an adult catheterization laboratory and 100 for a pediatric facility (there are fewer pediatric heart cases in general).

The procedure itself is straightforward, as we learned from Mr. Smith's case in Chapter 1. After a consent form has been signed, the patient is given a sedative or tranquilizer. Contrary to what many people believe, the patient remains awake during the procedure. After the patient is placed on a special X-ray cradle, the elbow and groin areas, where the catheters will enter, depending on the preference of the physicians, are cleansed with antibacterial solutions. Local anesthesia is injected into the skin that covers the targeted blood vessels. After the skin is deadened, there should be no further pain. Small incisions are made over the arteries and veins to be used, or alternatively, a direct puncture can be made through the skin. The long, thin catheters are then introduced over guide wires and advanced to the heart under fluoroscopic control. Once the catheters are there, the operator can record whatever pressures are necessary through the catheter, or inject a contrast agent into blood vessels or heart chambers via the catheter. There is surprisingly little discomfort during these injections, only a "hot flash" as the dye reaches the brain after circulating in the bloodstream. During these injections, a videotape recorder is turned on so that the catheterization team can play back the tape and note obstructions and other abnormalities. This helps to determine the angle to rotate the camera for subsequent injections. All injections are also recorded on 35-mm motion picture film. This will be the permanent record of the case, along with the graphic recordings of the pressure measurements. Once the catheterization procedure is complete, the patient is returned to his or her room for an overnight recovery period before being discharged the next day.

The decision to undergo coronary arteriography is made by the patient's physician in consultation with specialists and, of course, with the patient's consent. While coronary arteriography is the "gold standard" for documenting blockages in the coronary arteries, not all patients with prior heart attacks or suspected heart disease will be referred for this procedure. Often physicians feel they can adequately treat many patients who have few or mild symptoms without the need to define the coronary anatomy precisely; only when there is progressive pain will they refer patients for the procedure. This is a conservative-to-moderate approach. Physicians who take a moderate-to- aggressive approach look for features other than symptoms to help them make this decision: the abnormality of the exercise test, the radioisotopic studies, etc.

In summary, detection of heart disease can be made with a combination of history taking, physical examination and noninvasive testing (using the electrocardiogram and various types of stress tests). The coronary arteriogram, however, is still the only definitive way to make the diagnosis. Who should undergo this procedure? There is no "correct" answer. There are only guidelines to help physicians make decisions for those persons with symptoms, and for those persons suspected of having silent heart disease. Much of the final decision depends on how aggressive the physician is and how willing the patient is to undergo an invasive procedure.

CHAPTER

4

How Do Cigarettes and Cholesterol Lead to Blocked Arteries?

Cholesterol is the main part of the fatty deposits that block coronary arteries. The higher the blood level of one type of cholesterol (low-density lipoprotein, or LDL, cholesterol) the greater the likelihood blockages will occur. Damage to the blood vessel wall leads to the formation of these deposits, and this damage is accelerated by substances in cigarettes, by high blood pressure, and by diabetes.

It is April, 1953. There is a lull in the battle for Pork Chop Hill, the scene of one of the last battles in the stalemate known as the Korean War. As the American GIs pause to catch their breath, they break out their rations, including cans of pulverized "luncheon meats" full of meat and meat by-products with a high fat content. After the meal, another "macho"-male symbol appears: the cigarette. Meanwhile, in the nearby battalion aid stations, body bags are being prepared for their unfortunate buddies who were killed in the assault on the hill. Some of these men—those already dead and those soon to die—will be part of a study that will greatly influence the way physicians consider the relation between young people's eating and smoking habits and heart disease. The results of autopsies done on young American GIs killed in Korea will raise many questions about the harmful effects of the foods young people eat and the cigarettes they smoke. It is one thing to talk about risk factors in the abstract; it is another to see the opened blood vessels of young GIs filled with yellowish deposits of fat already beginning to block the channel of blood. How do these risk factors turn a normal heart into an abnormal heart?

THE NORMAL HEART

Simply stated, the heart is the body's pumping system for blood. It has its own "computer" to regulate the rate at which the heart must beat or contract in order to pump blood efficiently. Normally this rate is about 70 beats per minute for most of us, but during sleep it can slow down to the 40s, and during strenuous exercise approach 200. An essential part of the computer is the heart's pacemaker, a tiny sliver of specialized tissue located in the right atrium. As we noted in Chapter 3 when we discussed the electrocardiogram, it is here in the pacemaker tissue that the electric signal originates, and it is from here that it will spread throughout the rest of the heart. Once the electrical current reaches the level of an individual heart cell it depolarizes the outer lining of the cell. This allows chemical substances in the surrounding fluid to enter the cell. These agents, particularly calcium, act as catalysts for the contraction process. The energy for contraction comes from the oxidation (burning) of a sugar (glucose) in the presence of oxygen. All cells in the body operate in this fashion, though not all contract. Kidney cells, for example, may help in the filtering of body wastes, brain cells in thought processes, etc.; but all require an energy source (such as glucose or oxygen) in order to perform their specific actions.

How each cell "knows" what to do and how organs like the heart, brain and kidney have evolved from the microscopic union of one sperm cell and one egg cell are part of the mysteries of life—mysteries that are far more complex than the workings of the most advanced electronic computer. Suffice it to say that these organs *do* develop, each with its preordained purpose. The role of the heart is to pump blood with its precious cargo of oxygen and fuel sources to all the cells in the body. As long as the heart beats, the body lives. *If it stops for more than three minutes, vital functions in the brain will be irreparably harmed.*

The heart is actually composed of two pumps operating parallel to one another (Fig. A). The right collecting chamber (right atrium) collects blood from veins all over the body except

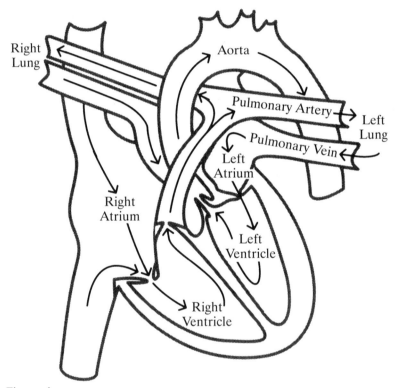

Figure A
General diagram of the heart: The right atrium receives "used" blood from the body, and the right ventricle pumps it through the pulmonary artery to the lungs to absorb fresh oxygen. The left atrium receives oxygenated blood from the lungs, and the left ventricle pumps it through the aorta to the rest of the body.

the lungs. This blood is "used" in the sense that it has been depleted of much of its oxygen. Somehow, new sources of oxygen have to be infused into it. Since we breathe air containing oxygen, the transfer of that oxygen to the blood stream must take place in the lung. The right atrium empties into the right ventricle, a pumping chamber that propels the blood through the pulmonary (lung) arteries so it can seep through the tiny air sacs at the end of the breathing tubules and collect the necessary oxygen. The blood reaches the lungs carrying only about 70% of the oxygen that it can hold; when it leaves the lungs (via the pulmonary veins) it is about 98% saturated. *The lungs represent the only system in the body where the draining vessels (the veins) have more oxygen than the entering vessels (the arteries).* The pulmonary veins bring the oxygenated blood to the left collecting chamber (the left atrium), which in turn empties into the left ventricle. This chamber is nearly 10 times thicker than the right ventricle and because the force of its contraction must propel the blood a great deal further than that of the right ventricle. The blood gushes out into the aorta, the main artery of the body, and through its many branches to the head, the limbs and the internal organs. The sequence of beating in the four chambers of the heart allows the collecting chambers to empty their blood into the ventricles first and then to fill while the ventricles pump. In both the collecting and pumping chambers, the right chambers contract a fraction of a second ahead of the left ones. All beats are controlled by the pacemaker and its accessory branches.

The size of the arterial vessels narrows considerably as they get closer to their final destination (the cell). The smallest level of blood vessels, the capillaries, are small enough to accommodate only a few red blood cells at a time and allow easy access to individual cells in an organ. As the oxygen and fuel sources diffuse out of the bloodstream into the cells, the waste products of cellular life diffuse into the blood from the cell. These waste products will eventually be blown off by the lungs (carbon dioxide) or excreted by the kidneys (nitrogenous wastes).

The heart muscle is performing a staggering task when it pumps blood continuously. Each heartbeat propels about two ounces of blood. If one calculates what the heart does in the typical life span of a 70-year-old person, the figures are astounding. Beating nearly 2.5 billion times, it will pump about 100 million gallons of blood throughout the body! As with all organ systems in the body, the heart itself needs nutrients. Immediately after the aorta begins its ascent from the left ventricle, it gives rise to two blood vessels that will supply the heart muscle with its own blood supply: the right and left coronary arteries (Fig. B). The right coronary artery supplies the right atrium and right ventricle and underside of the left ventricle; the left coronary artery supplies the rest of the left ventricle and the left atrium.

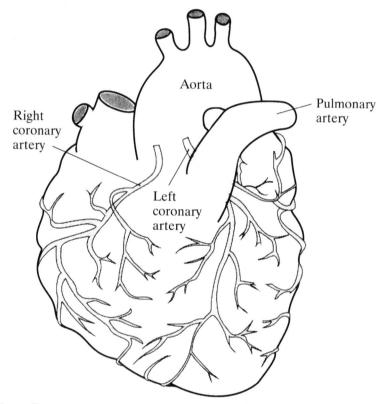

Figure B
The coronary circulation: Lying on the outer surface of the left ventricle are the major arteries that bring blood to the muscular walls of the heart.

These two main arteries have major branches that in turn have lesser branches. They are not wide vessels—the main coronary arteries are only about an eighth of an inch in diameter—but they are responsible for the health of the heart. The main vessels lie on the surface of the heart, like a crown—hence the name "coronary" derived from the Latin *corona*. The lesser branches penetrate the heart muscle itself.

THE ABNORMAL HEART

One of the fascinating features of coronary artery disease is that it is the main vessels (those lying on the surface of the heart) that develop blockages, not the vessels that dive deeply into the muscle layers. One theory is that the constant activity of the muscle as it contracts "massages" the deeper blood vessels and keeps their interiors clear. The other intriguing feature is that coronary veins do not develop blockages, only the arteries. There is a simpler explanation for this: The internal pressure in the veins is minimal compared to that in the arteries. We measure pressure as the height of a column of mercury. During contractions of the heart, it is usually 5–10 mm in the veins compared to 120–140 mm in the arteries. The higher the internal pressure, the greater the chance of damaging the lining of the blood vessel, which is one of the reasons blockages develop. Most blockages occur in the first third or so of a vessel's length; fortunately, the area can be reached with a special balloon catheter for dilatation, or widening (see Chapter 10). Since the more distal (distant) areas are relatively clear, they make excellent connecting points for the coronary bypass operation.

What do the blockages consist of? How did they get there? When we list the contents of the most common types of blockages we see a familiar word: cholesterol. Cholesterol in one or another of its forms is the main part of the *atheromatous plaque*, the scientific name for the blockage. *Athera* comes from the Greek; it means gruel or porridge. The plaques have a core that is quite soft and gruel-like. The other major component of the plaque is cellular. These cells lie around the central necrotic core and are mostly muscle cells, similar to those that normally form the middle layer of the vessel wall. What causes these cells to migrate from their normal position to the innermost lining of the vessel channel? We don't know. One important theory is the "response-to-injury" hypothesis proposed by Dr. Russell Ross and colleagues. They hypothesize that if the inner layer of the vessel wall is damaged in any way (by mechanical or chemical agents) small blood particles (platelets) stick to the tear and "patch it." They release chemical substances that attract the smooth muscle cells. If the injury is not repetitive, the defect can heal without plaque formation. With repeated injury, however (and some types of cholesterol themselves are believed to be capable of causing repeated injuries), the damage to the lining of the blood vessel is continuous. The healing process is never complete: Fatty substances accumulate, cellular debris is trapped within the gruel, and more and more smooth cells are attracted to the area. A plaque is formed. It grows, pushing out into the the lumen (or channel) of the vessel and narrowing the opening through which blood passes (Fig. C).

In animals, the major impetus to plaque formation following experimental injury to normal arteries is *sustained high levels of cholesterol in the blood.* High blood levels of cholesterol lead to further damage to the inner lining of the blood vessel—no matter what the initial cause of the internal injury—so that as the plaque builds, healing is prevented. A vicious cycle is perpetuated. The narrowed channel can lead to ischemia. When the channel is completely blocked—either by rupture of the plaque into the lumen or by a new blood clot full of platelets sitting on top of the plaque (Fig. C)—infarction (death of heart muscle) occurs.

The mechanism by which a new blood clot blocks an artery is under intensive investigation. Much of what we have learned from animal models can be only inferred for the human condition, not proven. It was not until cardiologists took a more active and aggressive stance against heart attacks that we learned more about complete blockages in humans. In 1982, Dr. Marcus DeWood reported that when cardiac catheterizations

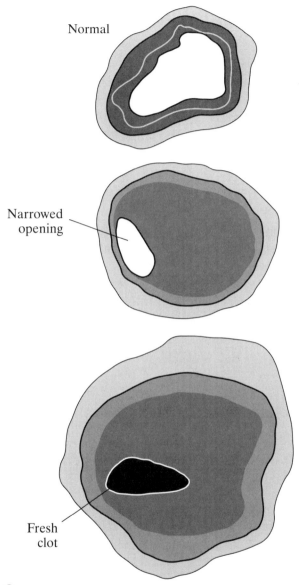

Figure C
Coronary arteries: Three cross sections of coronary arteries showing a
normal artery, one with a narrowed opening due to an accumulation of
fatty deposits, and one with an already narrowed opening that has been
"plugged" with a fresh clot.

were performed soon after patients were admitted to the hospital for a heart attack, a high percentage (90%) of completely occluded vessels were found. If patients were catheterized 12–14 hours later, the percentage of complete occlusions dropped to 54%. This suggested a platelet-filled clot had formed on a pre-existing plaque and then dissolved spontaneously and for unknown reasons. Furthermore, in patients dying of heart attacks after repeated bouts of severe angina, at autopsy the coronary arteries often showed evidence of sequential laying-down of clots. The final event was related to a fresh clot. These clots were made up of cellular debris and platelets. Findings such as these not only have important therapeutic implications, they also confirm our knowledge of the role of platelets in ischemia and infarction. Since one of the cheapest and most readily available anti-platelet agents is the ubiquitous aspirin tablet, a new era in cardiac therapy may be starting. The use of aspirin, and of drugs to break up clots once they have formed, is discussed in Chapters 10 and 11.

Veins, which are normally not the site of atherosclerosis, can be subject to that process only when they are also subjected to the blood pressure that is usually present in arteries. We see this, for example, when veins from the legs are used to bypass obstructed arteries in the heart. In time, the walls of the veins begin to resemble the walls of the arteries!

HOW DO THE RISK FACTORS ACTUALLY CAUSE HEART DISEASE?

Physicians, as well as lay people, have long been intrigued by why *cigarette smoking* increases the risk of cardiovascular disease. Do cigarettes do their damage through the products that are drawn into the lungs or through the products that are absorbed into the lining of the mouth? Are cigars and pipes as dangerous as cigarettes?

Cigarettes are made up of a multitude of products; probably the best known harmful components are tar and nicotine. However, about 90% of cigarette smoke consists of a dozen harmful *gases*. These include hydrogen cyanide, which can damage the lining of the lungs; nitrogen oxide, which robs the lungs of their elasticity and contributes to emphysema (loss of lung tissue); and carbon monoxide, which is associated with heart disease. The last gas is the same chemical substance that makes automobile exhaust fumes deadly!

Nicotine is another main culprit. This addictive plant compound produces a variety of changes inside the body. Nicotine stimulates the release of powerful hormones (catecholamines), which in turn stimulate the cardiovascular system. The best known of these hormones are adrenalin and related compounds; after a few puffs the smoker's heart will begin pounding an extra 15–25 beats per minute. Catecholamines also constrict small arteries throughout the body, elevating blood pressure by as much as 20 mm of mercury.

The combination of a faster heart rate and higher blood pressure causes the heart to work harder. When it works harder, it needs more oxygen. The trouble is that carbon monoxide reduces the oxygen supply. Because of certain chemical properties, carbon monoxide binds to the red blood cells more efficiently than oxygen. Thus, less oxygen is carried by the red blood cells to the cells of the body. Carbon monoxide also slows down the release of the remaining oxygen to the tissues. This may be one of the reasons that some smokers seem to have less energy and feel winded more often; in a sense they are not receiving an adequate oxygen supply throughout their bodies.

We see that the heart is affected by smoking in at least two ways: Nicotine raises the heart rate and blood pressure, and the heart is deprived of necessary oxygen by carbon monoxide. Carbon monoxide not only reduces the oxygen-carrying capacity of the blood, it also affects the circulatory system directly. The walls of the arteries become more permeable to substances like cholesterol which can then be deposited as crystals in the arterial walls. Smoking is also known to increase the clotting action in the blood, in part by acting on the platelets that patch a wounded area. As we have discussed, in arteries already narrowed by fatty deposits containing cholesterol, clotting of the platelets may form a plug that further blocks the artery and results in ischemia or a heart attack.

What about smoking and silent heart disease? Direct evidence of how cigarette smoking causes silent ischemia in patients with known heart disease was provided by Dr. John Deanfield and colleagues using Holter monitoring techniques described in Chapter 3. Cigarettes caused a marked reduction in blood flow to the heart in six out of eight patients tested!

Cigar and pipe smokers do *not* seem to have the same high risk for heart attacks as do cigarette smokers, probably because they do not inhale the smoke.

The ravages of *high blood pressure* on blood vessels throughout the body have been well documented by physicians for many years. Normal blood pressure is less than 140 mm when the heart is contracting (systolic pressure) and less than 90 mm when it is relaxed (diastolic pressure). Higher pressure causes damage to the arteries and capillaries; in the kidneys it leads to kidney failure; in the brain it leads to strokes; and in the heart to either coronary artery disease, direct weakening of the heart muscle, or both. High blood pressure may be one of the injurious stimuli that causes tears in the lining of blood vessels, thereby beginning the cycle of healing, injury, healing. It also can force more cholesterol compounds into the wall of the blood vessels, leading to plaque buildup. High blood pressure is particularly dangerous when combined with the vessel-damaging effects of cigarette smoking, or in the presence of high blood levels of cholesterol. But even alone, without the other risk factors, it can be a significant contributor to the atherosclerotic process. Once heart disease is present, the continued high blood pressure means the heart must work harder to pump blood against the increased resistance and is more likely to develop ischemia.

The role of *high blood levels of cholesterol* (above 240mg per 100 ml of blood) has already been alluded to. Cholesterol and its derivatives are found in great amounts in atherosclerotic plaques. One type of protein that is bound to cholesterol in the blood, called the low-density lipoprotein (or LDL) cholesterol, may actually cause vessel injury itself, as well as being a "carrier" to get the cholesterol into the vessel wall. If the LDL substance is the "bad guy" of the cholesterol world, then the high-density lipoprotein fraction (HDL) is the "good guy." This compound is protective in that it helps to transport cholesterol through the blood and back to the liver, where it can be broken down and excreted into the intestines. Much more remains to be learned about the interaction between LDL- and HDL-cholesterol, but one thing seems clear: You are better off with lower levels of LDL and higher levels of HDL! Unfortunately, there are not too many ways to raise HDL levels (regular exercise is one). Ways of reducing LDL levels are through diet and certain drugs (see Chapters 7 and 8).

The last major risk factor, *diabetes*, is often thought of by the public as simply "too much sugar in the blood," but it is a far more complex disease. While it is true that problems in the pancreas (the internal gland that produces insulin, the main regulator of body sugar) are responsible for the disease, we are not sure how to relate all of the complications of the disease to the blood sugar level, per se. Some problems are clearly related, especially the tendency for massive alterations in the composition of body fluids leading to coma and death. These complications can be prevented by insulin injections, and they no longer cause the deaths of diabetics, as they once did. Instead, diabetics die of cardiovascular disease—heart attacks, strokes and related problems.

The causes of the blood vessel disease in diabetics is not clear. There is considerable doubt that it is the blood sugar level, since well controlled diabetics seem to have about as many cardiovascular problems as poorly controlled ones. (This is still a controversial point, however, and we certainly recommend adequate insulin dosages for those persons that require them.) The longer the duration of the illness, the more cardiovascular complications the diabetic can expect. In the juvenile form—when the pancreas produces little or no insulin—the blood vessel complications are apt to be particularly troublesome by the middle years. On the other hand, in the adult-onset form, when the disease is not usually recognized until middle life, the pancreas still produces adequate amounts of insulin, but the insulin is "inefficient" for a variety of reasons. Cardiovascular complications are seen later in life in these adult-onset diabetics.

Unfortunately, the diabetic may not have the ability to control his or her destiny concerning cardiovascular disease—there are still too many unanswered questions about what causes the vascular problems. But it should be obvious to the reader that the other risk factors like smoking and high blood pressure can be controlled. There is simply no excuse for not doing so. Later in this book we will provide some helpful guidelines towards accomplishing those goals.

5

Can Stress Cause Heart Disease?
The Role of the "Mind-Body Connection"

How a person reacts to the stressful pressures and tensions of everyday life is the key to understanding how stress influences cardiovascular disease. Those persons who respond to stress with a greater release of certain hormones, body chemicals, and nervous system commands increase the chance of causing injury to their heart and blood vessels. This may be the physiologic basis for the role of what has been termed the "mind-body connection" in heart disease. Fortunately, physical exercise and mental relaxation blunt the effects of stress and, along with a reduction in certain coronary-prone personality traits (Type A behavior), can help fight heart disease.

In the movies and on television, it often seems that a heart attack usually occurs in a harried, overworked 60 year old executive who has just flown into a rage at one of his colleagues. Another popular variation is to have an attack occur during a heated argument with a family member. The message to the public is that somehow one or both of these stressful situations precipitated the heart attack. For many years physicians scoffed at this impression. We are now having second thoughts. Dr. James Muller of Harvard Medical School is one investigator who believes that there are a variety of factors that can "trigger" heart attacks and that "stress" can be one of them. We will discuss this more fully in Chapter 11, when we consider heart attacks in detail. In this chapter, we want to concentrate on stress itself. Does it play a role in the "mind-body connection" that Bill Moyers popularized in a 1993 PBS series, but to which many have alluded for years? What is stress, anyway?

Americans seem preoccupied with stress. Our whole lives are designed to avoid it! We look on the stereotypical laid-back person with a curiosity tinged with envy. Laid-back people seem more relaxed; the pressure and tension that are natural ingredients of work or interpersonal relationships don't appear to bother them as much as other people.

Many investigators believe that response to stress is the key to understanding the relationship betweeen stress and various types of disease. In other words, *it is not the pressure that is the problem, it's how the individual reacts to it that matters.* Some experts have pointed out the imbalance between various stressful stimuli in our environment (noise, pollution, physical exertion, marital problems, economic hardships, etc.) and our ability to cope with those stressful stimuli effectively.

Dr. Herbert Benson of Harvard Medical School (one of the earliest proponents of the "mind-body connection") defines stress as environmental conditions requiring behavorial adjustment. This idea conforms to the original medical concept conceived by Dr. Hans Seyle in the 1950s to emphasize that it is the *reaction* to the situation that causes the stress, rather than the physical, human, psychological, or psychosocial, conditions. Dr. Seyle also believed that disease states could be related to persistent stress.

Attempts to prove or disprove the Seyle hypothesis led to a number of interesting studies in the field of psychosomatic medicine. One of the most well known of these studies was the one reported by Drs. Thomas Holmes and Richard Rahl in 1967. They established an index for rating "life adjustment" based on a questionnaire. Marriage was the standard stress-causing event, nominally set at 50 units. The highest units were associated with death of a spouse, divorce, death of a close family member, or personal injury or illness. Scores based on these units were compared to sickness rates in over 500 men and women. The greater the stressful life changes (based on the scores), the greater likelihood of becoming ill. So although the concept of psychological factors affecting the body have often been discounted, the more medical research that is done, the more it emphasizes the concept of the mind-body connection. Even one's birthday can become an extra-risky time according to research presented at a 1993 cardiology meeting. Interestingly, married people have less illness than do widows or divorced people. Other studies also linked lack of social support to illness. The more extensive social, familial, and community contacts a person had, the less likely they were to die, at least during the course of the study.

What about job pressure? Is it an important factor? The affluent and educated seem less likely to develop cardiovascular disease than those in lower socioeconomic classes, who are also less educated. Are people who reach the top really exposed to less stress? Hardly, but they may well respond to it better. Maybe that's why they reached the top! Recent surveys show they may also have healthier living habits: not smoking, enjoying a good diet, being physically fit.

The most famous attempt to relate stress to heart disease was that of Drs. Meyer Friedman and Ray Rosenman, who described the Type A and Type B personalities and advanced the idea that the Type A personality was an independent risk factor for coronary artery disease. They defined the Type A personality as showing a constantly competitive attitude, even when challenges were nonexistent. Such a person cannot relax without feeling guilty about it! When pursuing a real challenge, the person is not only ambitious but inflexible in pursuit of the goal. At other times, the individual pursues several lines of thought at once. They frequently interrupt others, are constantly rushing through meals, are preoccupied with work, and are self-centered in interpersonal relationships. As a result of the latter, such relationships rapidly become unsatisfactory. Type A persons also can be observed tapping their feet, tensing their jaws, and exhibiting other signs of unnecessary muscular activity. Drs. Friedman and Rosenman felt that this behavorial syndrome was encouraged by the increasing urbanization and technological progress of contemporary society. People who can perform rapidly and aggressively get the special rewards. The Type B person, on the other hand, has no sense of urgency about work and doesn't have the personality traits just described—leading to a less stressful life and a lower risk of heart disease.

The reader may find this theory a bit too pat to accept at face value—many physicians shared the same skepticism when it was first proposed. What made the medical profession sit up and take notice was the result of an eight-and-a-half year follow-up study of over 3100 men that Drs. Friedman and Rosenman and their colleagues reported in 1976. They found that Type A men were twice as likely as Type B men to develop coronary artery disease. This study, the Western Collaborative Group Study, appeared to be confirmed by psychosocial data from the Framingham Study, which also extended the conclusions to women. There are even recent studies showing that a relationship exists between Type A behavior and the degree of blockages on the coronary arteriograms. However, these theories also have their debunkers. The reason is that other prospective studies, similar in design to the Western Collaborative Group Study, have not supported the importance of Type A behavior as an independent risk factor. Also even more recent coronary arteriographic studies have refuted the conclusions of the earlier "positive" studies. What can we make of this confusion?

First, we must keep in mind that accurate measurement of Type A behavior is not easy. A self-reporting questionnaire is not as reliable as a structured, personal interview conducted by a trained observer. Second, the timing of the interview is crucial. You can't expect to interview someone just before a major procedure (like bypass surgery) or right after a heart attack and expect to observe a person's usual (baseline) personality traits. Other factors—age, sex, smoking history, etc.—must also be taken into account. Whether or not the subject has ever had a coronary event is especially important. We have seen in Chapters 3 and 4 that conventional wisdom about risk factors assigns a much greater importance to their effect on initial events. After such an event, the patients may modify risk factors (and behavior), making conclusions about causative factors dubious.

Even with the controversy about a "global" Type A pattern unresolved, can there still be a good case made for the importance of *certain* personality traits leading to coronary events? Dr. C.D. Jenkins (inventor of the Jenkins Activity Survey) has provided data to support the view that anxiety and coronary artery disease appear to be related since hostility and repressed anger are features that occur over and over in coronary patients. Dr. Redford Williams of Duke University has been particularly impressed with these two factors and has considered them the most important of the behavioral abnormalities.

Is there any way of unifying what we know about the physiologic mechanisms of heart disease with psychosocial or emotional factors? Can stress cause heart disease to develop? Can it aggravate pre-existing heart disease?

During periods of stress, the body releases certain hormones into the bloodstream. Along with impulses from the nervous system, these hormones help regulate various essential activities of the body including speeding up the heart rate, making the heart beat more forcefully, and constricting the blood vessels to help propel the stream of blood. This reaction is ideally suited for physical exertion because it serves to make the body a more efficient machine. The hormones also stimulate the release of sugars and fats from storage deposits in the liver to fuel this machinery. In early history, such reactions could be essential for survival. Properly fueled and with all systems ready, one had the necessary stamina to either engage an enemy in battle or flee— whichever the circumstances dictated. But in modern times, this "fight or flight" reaction may not be so beneficial. If an individual has no one to fight, or run from, then all these excess chemicals being poured into the bloodstream may have deleterious effects on the heart and blood vessels.

Disruption of the internal layers in the blood vessel wall may result from the intense constriction of muscle cells caused by the stress-released hormones. An increase in blood clotting substances can also occur as a result, which in turn can lead to clot formation on the injured interior of the blood vessel. As we discussed in Chapter 4, constant or repetitive injury may cause permanent damage to the vessel wall in some individuals. In others, the wall will repair itself. Add an additional vascular insult—such as the harmful agents in cigarettes—to the tense, anxious executive, and it is a set-up for trouble. The damage does *not* have to occur at the time of emotional argument, but events can be set in motion by the stressful incident. These harmful effects of emotional stress were dramatically emphasized during the Iraqi missile attacks on Israel during the Persian Gulf War. The number of heart attacks in frightened elderly people increased significantly.

Most of what we have discussed is how stress leads to the development of obstruction in the blood vessel. Unfortunately, though, there is no formula to explain the relative contributions of stress, high blood pressure, smoking, cholesterol, etc. Experiments on animals kept under a great deal of stress show that they develop blockages more quickly than similarly fed but non-stressed animals. We also know that the cholesterol level in humans can be influenced by stressful circumstances. Students' cholesterol levels are higher before exams, for example. Wouldn't it be nice if we also had data that showed a direct relationship between a stressful event and transient heart damage? Thanks to studies with the Holter monitor that were cited earlier in the book, we now have such data.

Even prior to these Holter studies showing ischemia, Dr. Bernard Lown and associates at the Harvard School of Public Health demonstrated that mental arithmetic in patients could bring about both mild and severe ventricular arrhythmias. They also performed experiments on animals who were psychologically stressed by the use of electric shocks at feeding time. In these animals, potentially fatal arrhythmias could be induced much more easily under stressed conditions than under non-stressed conditions. As a result of these experiments, part of Dr. Lown's approach to treating arrhythmias involves psychological counseling as well as medication.

Because the impulse to trigger the "fight or flight" syndrome can be mental as well as physical, is it possible that some people with certain personality traits expose themselves to an accelerated development of coronary artery blockage and/or irregular heart beats because of the stress they experience when reacting to their environment? This is a real possibility. How does one avoid it?

We realize that coping with the challenges of the world is not an easy task, but half the battle is in realizing that inner stress and tension relate to how the challenge is perceived rather than to the challenge itself. Guidelines for reducing stress in one's life don't have to be complex. They can include physical relaxation brought on, paradoxically, by a strenuous event such as jogging. We believe very strongly that the beneficial effects that exercise has on the body enable a person to cope better with the stressful pressures and tensions they encounter in daily life. Chapter 9 describes these beneficial effects which include lowering of the heart rate and blood pressure in more detail. Thus, proper cardiovascular conditioning achieved through an exercise program helps to blunt the deleterious actions of certain body chemicals and nervous system commands that are present in stressful situations.

Dr. Benson and others advocate mental relaxation techniques, but even simple things like enjoying one's work and free time can be helpful. When simple measures fail, stress reduction techniques are available, either in courses or with individual therapists. (More about this in Chapter 12.) Although degrees of stress and severity of psychological problems are hard to measure scientifically, we cannot ignore the studies that illustrate the importance of the mind's effect on the workings of the body. It is also important to note that a person who has a chronic illness such as heart disease, always feels *some* type of psychological stress. This factor is also discussed further in Chapter 12.

Can stress reduction really have an effect on heart disease? A growing number of cardiologists think so. Dr. Friedman and associates published data in 1986 showing that when individuals with Type A personalities received special behavorial counseling to reduce their Type A activity, they had almost 50% fewer recurrent heart attacks or other cardiac events than Type As who received only conventional group counseling. Whether the results of this conversion to non-Type A pattern are independent of changes in other risk factors is still unclear, but the bottom line is that reducing the effects of physical and mental stress is a worthwhile goal in the fight against heart disease. It also helps in better enjoying one's life—a worthwhile goal in itself.

6

The Outlook for Patients with Heart Disease

Unfortunately, only half the population with heart disease will have angina as the first clinical symptom; the rest will either die suddenly or have a non-fatal heart attack without ever having any warning signs. Once heart disease has developed, the most important factors in determining the outlook for a patient are the number of vessels with critical blockages and the pumping ability of the left ventricle. This is true for both painful and silent heart disease.

Mist shrouds the fjords as the jetliner makes its final descent. Suddenly, the sun breaks through, and the beauty of the Norwegian landscape is revealed below. Mountains and rivers quickly blend into the typically urban setting of Oslo, Norway. This city is where a remarkable study is underway, a study using ordinary, healthy white-collar workers as its subject—ordinary in every sense but one, that is. These healthy workers have been found to have severe but totally asymptomatic coronary artery disease. Data about what has happened to them—and what continues to happen to them—will affect every one of us in Western societies.

This important study is being undertaken at a time when silent heart disease is finally being realized as a public health issue. Yet, mortality due to heart disease is definitely falling in most Western countries. Is there some contradiction here? Not necessarily. In fact, if we can now learn to treat silent heart disease effectively, we may well see another and even sharper drop in cardiovascular mortality.

Death from heart attacks and related events hit their peak in the early 1960s and has fallen off at about 3% per year since then. Unfortunately, cardiovascular disease is still the number one cause of death, with cancer second. The fall in cardiovascular mortality can be attributed to two factors: better control of coronary risk factors to prevent disease and better treatment of the disease once found. Most physicians would agree with the epidemiologic specialists in our schools of public health that it is the former feature, rather than the latter, that is *most* responsible for this decline. In other words, despite all our technological advances in medical and surgical treatment, it is probably correct to suggest that *fewer people are dying from cardiovascular disease because fewer people are developing cardiovascular disease in the first place.* That is why emphasizing the role of healthy living habits in preventing disease is one of the major purposes of this book. We must also consider, however, those individuals already afflicted. For them, control of risk factors is still important, but so is treatment. What do we know about their prognosis? When will they develop heart attacks? When will they die? What effect does silent ischemia have on their longevity?

It would be nice to think that the course of a person with heart disease would follow a natural progression. A "natural" progression means there should be an asymptomatic or presymptomatic phase in which the person has partial blockage of the coronary arteries but has not yet progressed to the point where symptoms have yet developed. In this "natural" order the next step would be the development of chest pain (angina), which we hope would be treated. Some years later, a heart attack would occur, and perhaps another one some time later. The patient would either recover or die from the acute or chronic effects of the heart attacks. While this simplistic schema does occur in some individuals, it would be foolish to think that heart disease in most patients behaves in this way. *Fully half of all patients with coronary artery disease either die of their disease or have a non-fatal heart attack without ever having experienced "warning" chest pains.* When autopsies are performed on these victims (or coronary arteriograms on the more fortunate survivors), the extent and severity of their heart disease is often striking. This is why many investigators believe that transient heart damage is probably occurring during the asymptomatic phase—even though this goes against the "natural" progression taught for so many years in our medical schools!

Heart attacks or death can occur at any time in a person with heart disease, but there are certain features of the vessel blockages that make it more likely. One of these is the number of vessels involved. As we have seen in Chapter 3, there are two main coronary arteries, the right and the left. Actually, since the left coronary artery quickly divides into two major branches, we usually consider the human heart to have three major arteries: the right and the two left arteries (called the left anterior descending and left circumflex arteries).

Early in the 1970s, a series of reports from several major medical centers in the United States established unequivocally that a critical blockage* of the main left coronary artery was the single most important blockage, the one that had the most negative effect on prognosis. Following diagnosis of this type of blockage by coronary arteriography, chances of surviving five years are under 50%. These figures are explained by the fact that no other single blockage can cause so much damage when a complete occlusion finally occurs. A large portion of the left

---

*A critical blockage narrows the vessel lumen by at least 70%. This can be measured by the coronary arteriogram as well as at autopsy.

ventricle will be severely damaged, if not killed outright. The immediate consequences include not only a fatal irregularity of the heart beat (which can even occur with occlusion of less important vessels) but also a severe reduction in the pumping ability of the heart as a result of the massive insult to the main pumping chamber. Occlusions of the main right coronary artery usually cause far less damage. Only a combination of blockages in all three major coronary arteries rivals a blockage in the main left coronary artery in destructive power. Blockages in all three vessels (called "three-vessel" or "triple-vessel" disease) is, therefore, another almost equally bad prognostic finding. Mortality from two-vessel disease is less that from three-vessel disease. Finally, mortality is least when only one vessel is involved (unless it is the main left artery). Within the one-vessel category, disease of the left anterior descending coronary artery (the most important branch of the main left coronary artery) carries the worst outlook, but this may be only about 15% mortality five years after diagnosis.

The other major contributing feature to survival is the pumping ability of the left ventricle. As that ability diminishes, mortality increases. If there is only a small region of scar in the left ventricle, survival will hardly be influenced. A larger scar or out-pocketing (called an aneurysm) does have a negative effect, however; when there is more dead or poorly functioning muscle than normally functioning muscle, the outlook can be dismal. For example, with widespread and severe scarring of the heart, five-year survival will be only 30% and 10-year survival 15%.

As discussed in Chapter 7, survival can be influenced in a positive way when patients with coronary artery disease control risk factors, especially cigarette smoking—but again one must consider the underlying anatomy. When there are extensive blockages or severe left ventricular dysfunction, it requires more than control of risk factors alone to cause increased survival. This is where aggressive medical and surgical therapy must be employed. These techniques are especially important during the early stages of a heart attack or when the anginal pattern has progressed so rapidly that angina at rest is common (the so-called unstable angina or pre-infarction syndrome).

When medical and surgical therapy is employed, the natural history of these disorders can be modified. As will be discussed in Chapter 10, the role of coronary artery surgery is especially dramatic in patients with left main disease, those with three-vessel disease, and those with poor left ventricular function. This was determined by three large-scale randomized trials, the Veterans Administration Cooperative Trial and the Coronary Artery Surgery Study (CASS), both performed in the United States, and the European Coronary Surgery Study.

In all syndromes of heart disease, one of the most feared complications is a fatal irregularity (arrhythmia) of the heart beat, termed ventricular fibrillation. Other arrhythmias are not fatal, but this one is because the ventricular beating is very rapid, uncoordinated and *ineffectual*. Whether inside or outside the hospital, this (not a simple stopping of the heart) is the terminal event in the overwhelming number of patients, though both events are called "cardiac arrests." Sometimes ventricular fibrillation can be corrected with an electrical countershock to the patient's chest. Best results occur when a properly equipped cardiopulmonary resuscitation (CPR) team is present. In a hospital, such a team can respond to a "cardiac arrest" page within minutes. The fatal rhythm can often be halted, at least temporarily, in many victims. Outside of the hospital, the appearance of such a team within the three minutes or so before death or irreversible brain damage occurs is, of course, a rarity. This is why a bystander who took a CPR course and is properly trained in closed-chest cardiac massage procedures can be of great help. By massaging the heart and at least preserving some circulation, more time is bought for the arrival of the cardiopulmonary resuscitation team.

Many times the forerunner of ventricular fibrillation is ventricular tachycardia, an arrhythmia that often responds to drugs and is not necessarily fatal. Techniques to detect ventricular tachycardia in patients with heart disease include exercise tests, Holter monitoring and sophisticated electrophysiological studies in the cardiac catheterization laboratory. One of the exciting aspects of studying these rhythm irregularities is finding out how closely they can be related to emotional upsets and other non-cardiac nervous system factors, as Dr. Lown's group has reported. Although ventricular arrhythmias are most common in patients with heart disease, they can also affect those with normal hearts. Fortunately, these unexplained deaths do not represent the same public health hazards as those related to silent coronary artery disease.

We know a considerable amount about the outlook for patients with known coronary artery disease; do we know as much about asymptomatic patients with silent heart disease? Quite frankly, no. We do have some information, however, that we can compare to what is known about symptomatic heart disease.

We know that once a person has survived a painful heart attack for at least a year, the yearly mortality is reported at about 4–5%. This is an average figure—there will be variations based on the number of diseased vessels and the state of left ventricular function, as discussed earlier. How does this compare to someone who has had a silent, or unrecognized, heart attack? This is, of course, an electrocardiographic diagnosis, pure and simple. Evidence that the damage is there and wasn't on a previous electrocardiogram taken a month or a year earlier. We have noted that data from the Framingham Study and other centers indicate that about 25% of all heart attacks fit this picture, even allowing for cases of "indigestion" that might have escaped medical attention when they occurred. The Framingham investigators are impressed by these figures.

"At first, I was surprised," said Dr. William Kannel of the Boston University Medical Center (and former medical director of the Framingham Study) when we spoke to him. "Despite the fact that people in Framingham had become very much aware of our study because of the publicity attached to it, and were inclined to be very sensitive to any episode of chest discomfort, no matter how insignificant, the incidence of silent heart attacks in 1980 remained at the same level it had been in 1970, about 25%."

But was the disorder more benign than a painful heart attack? "According to our follow-up data, the outlook is the same!" Dr. Kannel's findings involving 213 patients with silent heart attacks and 718 patients with painful ones were reported in 1984. The reader will be quick to realize that, in actuality, the outlook may be worse for an unrecognized heart attack since the victim must first survive it to have it "detected" on the next routine electrocardiogram!

What of prognosis in silent ischemia? Follow-up studies are available in all three types of silent ischemia. In Type 1 patients, those who are totally asymptomatic, the most detailed study has come from Dr. Jan Erikssen at the University of Oslo in Norway. In Chapter 3 we learned that after screening 2014 middle-aged men, first with exercise tests and then with coronary arteriography when appropriate, Dr. Erikssen and colleagues identified 50 patients with one or more blockages in their coronary arteries. Eight years after the study began, there were three deaths, two of them in patients with three-vessel disease. By the 15-year mark, there were 14 deaths, 8 in the three-vessel disease group. This works out to about a 3% per year mortality in these latter patients, a chilling statistic.

We asked Dr. Erikssen about these six deaths. "Most developed angina before their death, but some died suddenly. Several had a massive infarction. Nearly all of those in the three-vessel group who are still alive have either developed cardiac symptoms or had a progression of disease on their repeat coronary arteriograms."

In the Type 2 patients, those with a previous heart attack, there is also data from several centers showing that when silent ischemia is detected on exercise testing in certain patients after a heart attack, the outlook is not good. These high-risk patients are those who have extensive disease and reduced function of the heart. Brand new data also show the importance of silent ischemia on Holter monitoring in patients after heart attacks. Patients with evidence of silent ischemia—whether or not they had symptoms—had a much higher incidence of future cardiac events than those without silent ischemia. One of these reports came from the same group of Johns Hopkins Medical Center investigators that had previously reported a similar study dealing with patients who had painful as well as silent angina (Type 3 in our classification). Using Holter monitors to record the frequency and duration of episodes of silent ischemia, these physicians startled the medical world with their 1986 report showing the drug treatment of unstable angina was not necessarily successful just because the symptoms had remitted! Silent ischemia on the Holter monitor was associated with over a 40% incidence of worsening of symptoms in the 30-day follow-up period. These included heart attacks or the need for emergency coronary surgery procedures. By contrast, patients recovering from unstable angina without silent ischemia only had about a 10% incidence of such events. In 1987 they published the two-year follow up. This remarkable pattern had persisted!

All in all, these reports on the outlook for patients with coronary artery disease emphasize the need to look beyond symptoms for indications of how well patients will do in the future. Silent ischemia is the newest of these prognostic markers and one about which the general public will continue to hear more in the years ahead. There are other markers as well; not all are related to active ischemia. For example, it is well established that even in the absence of active ischemia (painful or silent) a heart that has been extensively damaged by previous heart attacks and has poor cardiac function is in deep trouble. We have commented on this earlier in discussing the importance of left ventricular function as well as the danger of certain types of irregular heart beats that can lead to sudden death outside the hospital.

Sudden death remains one of the most feared endpoints in patients with coronary artery disease, especially when it occurs outside the hospital and emergency rescue squads are not readily available. It is estimated that 250,000–350,000 Americans die in this manner every year. While the definition of sudden death varies, it is generally accepted as death within a short period (often one hour or less, but sometimes within 24 hours of the patient's collapse). As expected, when these patients are examined at autopsy, almost all show evidence of coronary artery disease. A much smaller number have valvular disease or heart muscle disease; rarely, no structural abnormalities at all are present. When coronary artery disease is present, it is extensive.

The noted cardiac pathologist, Dr. William Roberts, and his associates at the National Institutes of Health have published a series of reports over the last decade on the number of fatty deposits that are present in the coronary arteries of people dying in and out of hospitals. In one of these studies, reported in 1981, they dealt only with sudden death and compared the autopsy findings in a group of persons with known coronary artery disease to those who were apparently healthy. At this point, it will probably not surprise the reader to learn that the extent of fatty deposit and of near and total blockage was remarkably similar in the two groups! Scars of prior heart attacks were also common in the "healthy" patients!

About 50,000 persons per year die suddenly and without prior symptoms. With so much disease present at death, one could reasonably wonder if they weren't having some ischemic episodes prior to their death. The scars of unrecognized heart attacks provide some evidence that they were. We can also surmise that many of them may have had silent ischemia as well, but obviously this is harder to prove in a retrospective manner once someone is dead. However, from Dr. Erikssen's study in Norway, we do know that some patients with silent ischemia, followed prospectively, will die suddenly before developing overt symptoms. Similarly, there are some fascinating reports—not all of them published, unfortunately—of patients who are resuscitated from sudden death and transported to hospitals for treatment. In the course of their workup to find the cause of their sudden death, coronary arteriograms usually reveal extensive coronary disease. With appropriate testing, silent ischemia has been documented in previously "healthy" survivors; a good example includes nine such individuals in Minneapolis. More cases are needed, however, before we can fully confirm the hypotheses linking silent ischemia and sudden death in apparently healthy people.

In conclusion, we have seen how some clues to survival in persons with coronary artery disease can be gleaned from knowledge of the heart's anatomy, which can be determined by coronary arteriography, and by a knowledge of the heart's pumping ability, which can be obtained from both invasive and non-invasive means. Because of the technological advances in noninvasive testing, especially the echocardiogram (a device using ultrasound waves) and radionuclide procedures, heart function can be adequately studied in many patients without the need for cardiac catheterization. A 1992 study from the Lown group claimed that over half of all cardiac catheterizations are unnecessary. Even if this figure is exaggerated, many patients with stable symptoms and good exercise tolerance can be successfully treated without catheterization. There is no question that regardless of the technique employed to document cardiac function, important information is obtained. In general, the poorer the heart's pumping ability, the worse the outlook. There are always exceptions, however. Some individuals with normal heart function will die in the next hour, and some with very weakened hearts will live for the next decade.

Because of this uncertainty in predicting cardiovascular mortality (unlike, for example, the much greater certainty of death once cancer has spread throughout the body), we always emphasize the positive in talking to patients with coronary artery disease, even with advanced disease. New therapies and new procedures are always emerging. Physicians never give up, nor should the patient. On the other hand, *because things seem to be going well, don't lower your guard.* This book has cited several examples of individuals who thought their hearts were sound, but weren't, and of others who had a heart attack and thought they were over the worst, but weren't. All these people were misled because heart disease can be a silent killer as well as a painful one. *In the battle against heart disease, take nothing for granted.* Even if the physician is complacent, the medical "consumer" should not be!

CHAPTER

7

Preventing Heart Disease by Correcting Risk Factors

Primary prevention means preventing heart disease in healthy persons. *Secondary prevention* means preventing further heart damage in persons with known heart disease. New data shows that lowering blood cholesterol levels with diet and drugs can help accomplish these goals. Other studies show the beneficial effects on cardiovascular disease when other risk factors are corrected. Methods to stop smoking and control high blood pressure have also proven to be effective.

The American news media had a field day in the summer of 1986 when a youngster from California turned in her parents to the local police "for their own good" because she had observed them using drugs. While visions of a new era of child informers (as in George Orwell's novel *1984*) sent shivers down some of our spines, others of us were not so sure that it was such a bad idea. After all, the drugs were not only illegal, they were harmful. Perhaps this is what was necessary to get the parents off the stuff! In the end (or what is hoped will be the end), the parents were rehabilitated and reunited with their daughter. It would be stretching the point a bit to say that this might also be an effective way to stop cigarette smoking—after all, the butts are *not* illegal—but in terms of body injury, cigarette smoking certainly has a far more widespread, deleterious effect on more people than does drug addiction! There are an estimated 60 million cigarette smokers in the United States today. Untold numbers will contract cardiovascular disease as a result of this habit, not to mention the hundreds of thousands who will succumb to lung cancer and other respiratory diseases. Maybe they should be "turned in" to a "health police" unit for their own good! If not, how do we get them to stop smoking? That and other issues in the control of coronary risk factors is what this chapter is all about.

People often ask if they can do anything to prevent heart disease. If, indeed, people want to lower their chances of developing heart disease, the most important change of behavior or lifestyle would have to be described as learning to do things in moderation. What does that mean? One doesn't have to run marathons, give up a New York sirloin forever, deny oneself the desserts offered at a daughter's wedding or an anniversary dinner at the best restaurant in town. It also doesn't mean that because you are a foreman on a construction project or a Wall Street broker that you must quit your stressful job. Unfortunately, many people assume such extremes are necessary when they read or hear that their current lifestyle could create serious heart problems. They assume that the kind of measures that must be taken in order to lower their risk of developing heart disease would be overwhelming. Because of this defeatist (or fatalistic) attitude, they decide not to try to modulate their behavior at all!

In previous chapters, we learned about the major risk factors: what they are and how they are harmful. Now we'll see what you can do about them. Don't panic and think you have or will develop heart disease because you've gained five pounds on a holiday! Each risk factor—in small amounts—will not be likely to cause you trouble. However, if you have appreciable amounts of one or more risk factors, you need to be careful and consider changing your lifestyle.

The body of evidence linking certain risk factors to the development of heart attacks is overwhelming. Hence, any program to prevent heart attacks *must* include detailed plans to control these risk factors. As discussed in Chapter 3, the risk factors are high blood cholesterol, cigarette smoking, diabetes, high blood pressure (hypertension) and, to a lesser degree, obesity.

Control of risk factors is not just for people with known heart disease; in fact, a large body of opinion—with which we agree—argues that control of these risk factors is probably more important in people without known heart disease. *Primary prevention* (that is, preventing disease from developing in persons not known to have disease) may, therefore, be more beneficial than *secondary prevention* (control of risk factors in patients already experiencing heart problems in order to prevent further problems). In other words, once the proverbial horse is out of the barn, closing the barn door may have no value. We do believe it has *some* value in preventing further development of heart disease, but not as much as maintaining good health habits in early life.

How to control your diet to lower cholesterol is the subject of an extensive discussion in Chapter 8 (with heart-healthy recipes provided at the end of the book) and will not be discussed at length here, but we will highlight some of the medical trials that show the value of lowering blood cholesterol to more normal levels. The most important of these were completed so recently that none of the books on heart disease that are currently available to the general public—and that we surveyed in preparing for our book—include all of this data.

In the area of primary prevention, the National Institutes of Health in Bethesda, Maryland (through the division on Heart, Blood and Lung Diseases) conducted a mammoth screening program across the United States. This was the Lipid Research Clinics Primary Prevention Trial. Beginning in 1973, 12 clinics in this trial recruited 3806 middle-aged men (35–59 years old) whose serum cholesterol levels were in the range usually associated with a higher than average risk of developing heart attacks (levels above 265 mg%, which means more than 265 mg per each 100 ml of blood). This is the top 5% of cholesterol levels for this age group in the United States. Nearly half a million men were screened from 1973–1976 to recruit the study group. Men with definite heart disease, abnormal resting electrocardiograms, or high blood pressure were excluded. All the men were placed on moderate cholesterol-lowering diets. They were then randomly assigned to additional treatment with either a specific cholesterol-lowering agent (cholestyramine—trade name Questran—which binds cholesterol in the intestine and causes it to be excreted in the stool) or a placebo (an inactive agent packaged in a similar manner to that of the active drug).

The average period of follow-up was nearly 7.5 years (range 7–10). The study was terminated in the summer of 1983 and its results were reported in 1984. Results showed that addition of the drug lowered the cholesterol level more than the placebo (42 mg% versus 4 mg%). This was not unexpected, but what was particularly encouraging was that along with the fall in blood cholesterol went a fall in serious cardiac events (heart attacks and death). There were 155 such events with the active drug compared to 187 with the placebo. This represents what statisticians call a "significant" finding—in other words, an important reduction, not one attributed to chance. This was the first scientifically valid study that could make this point. All previous studies—and there had been many—had been flawed by inappropriate methods either in randomizing the patients or in analyzing the data. In some valid studies (such as the Oslo Heart Study), other risk factors were controlled, as well as cholesterol levels. This will be discussed further later. Suffice it to say that the Lipid Research Clinics study represents a landmark.

In 1985, shortly after the publication of the Lipid Research Clinics study, another study in a much smaller number of persons appeared with equally important results. However, this study dealt with secondary prevention—the patients in the study group had already shown evidence of coronary artery disease (angina or heart attacks). This was the National Institutes of Health Type II Coronary Intervention Study and included 116 patients, all on low-fat, low-cholesterol diets. They were again randomized to either cholestyramine or a placebo, and once more the lowering of the cholesterol levels in those receiving cholestyramine was impressive (26% versus 5% in the placebo group). Instead of looking at an endpoint of heart attacks or deaths, this study looked at progression of disease as determined by sophisticated analysis of coronary arteriograms. Progression was much less in the cholestyramine group than in the placebo group. This study—and one reported in 1987 in coronary bypass patients—illustrates why we believe that even after the horse has left the barn, there may still be some value in shutting the door! It's never too late to lower your blood cholesterol level.

All these studies reinforce the importance of a low cholesterol level—even for persons who have already been told by their doctors not to worry because their levels are "average" for their age. This is a fallacy! As with blood pressure, so with cholesterol: the lower, the better! These studies also confirm the earlier epidemiological studies cited in Chapter 3 that showed that persons maintaining a lower cholesterol level (due to low-fat diets without drugs) had less chance of developing heart disease. What is an acceptable level in Western society? We believe it is less than 200 mg%. These studies were the first to reliably show that lowering cholesterol levels prevents heart attacks in healthy people or progression of coronary artery disease in patients with known heart disease. They explain the importance of active intervention in risk modification. Cholestyramine is not the only drug that can be used. Research is under way in several centers involving patients who have been placed on other kinds of cholesterol-lowering drugs.

Other examples of how successful a risk modification policy is can be found in studies leading to control of two other major risk factors: cigarette smoking and high blood pressure. Once the cigarette habit has taken hold, all is not lost! There is ample evidence that quitting helps. In fact, the risk of a smoker experiencing a future heart attack decreases to that of a non-smoker *within 5 to 10 years of quitting*. This is based on data from the Framingham Study, from a Kaiser Permanente Hospital study of

26,000 people, and the Oslo Heart Study that was mentioned earlier. Techniques for quitting smoking vary. Hypnosis, group therapy, drugs—whatever is required should be used.

In 1986, the American College of Physicians' Health and Public Policy Committee made a series of recommendations to help people stop smoking. They did so not only because of the risks of developing heart disease, but because cigarette smoking has been implicated as a "causal or facilitating factor" in other diseases as well. These diseases include lung cancer, bladder cancer, emphysema, chronic bronchitis and other types of vascular disease besides coronary artery disease such as stroke, circulatory problems in the legs, etc. The committee's report had some interesting statistics based on surveys of smokers' attitudes. Ninety percent of smokers would like to quit smoking and about 15% actually attempt to stop their habit each year. Many are successful, and two-thirds of those who are able to quit do so entirely on their own. There is so much pressure on smokers to quit—familial attitudes, anti-smoking laws, warnings about dire health consequences—that it is expected that in the future even more smokers will be able to quit and not return to smoking. It is the long-term abstinence rates that remain a problem. "Relapse" rates of 70–80% one year after stopping were not uncommon in the mid-1970s, but by the early 1980s, they had dropped to 40–50%, a somewhat encouraging sign.

What techniques can physicians recommend to their patients that will help them stop smoking and continue their abstinence? Smoking is both physically and psychologically addicting, and smoking cessation techniques must address both problems. There are five major smoking cessation techniques: (1) drug therapy, (2) behavior modification, (3) educational and commercial programs, (4) hypnosis, and (5) multiple risk factor reduction programs.

Drug therapy consists of three types of agents, but two of these—smoking deterrents and vegetable-based products that serve as a substitute for cigarettes—have not been widely used and are not very successful. The third type of agent is a nicotine-containing smoking substitute. The first such substitute used was lobeline, but this was found to be no better than a placebo. A nicotine gum, Nicorette, showed more promise and was approved by the Food and Drug Administration (FDA) in 1984 after studies of the drug (when it was combined with extensive counseling) apparently showed a significant advantage over placebos. Because there are cardiovascular effects related to chewing the gum (it releases nicotine), the drug is not advisable for patients with heart disease or high blood pressure. The gum appears particularly useful in overcoming withdrawal symptoms while the ex-smoker participates in a behavior modification program.

A *behavior modification program* can consist of a variety of techniques emphasizing self-control, contingency management and adverse conditioning. An element of self-monitoring is key. Common *contingency management* features include "contracts" for reward and punishment; for example, after abstaining for a designated period of time, the person rewards him- or herself by purchasing a much desired item of clothing or taking a weekend trip. The committee recommended several good self-help guides: the "Smokers Self-Testing Kit" (Public Health Service publication #1904) from the Office on Smoking and Health of the Department of Health and Human Services, Washington, D.C.; "A Lifetime of Freedom from Smoking" from the American Lung Association, New York City; "Quit for Good" from the National Cancer Institute, Bethesda, Maryland; and the "I Quit Kit" from the American Cancer Society, New York City (the latter is summarized later in the chapter). The *adverse conditioning programs* include electroshock (rather drastic, even for this unhealthy habit, so it's only used as a last resort in those individuals agreeing to try it), sensory deprivation (lying in bed in a quiet, dark room for a day) and satiation treatments (smoke double or triple the amount usually smoked in a short period, until nauseated). The adverse conditioning studies resulted in a 76% abstinence rate over a six-year period in one study, though most experts still feel a combination of a self-management program, a contingency management program and adverse conditioning offers the best approach to behavior modification.

Education is often used in combination with behavior modification and other anti-smoking methods. All of the official organizations cited earlier have educational materials available, plus providing lecturers for groups. Physicians can also join in this process. Smoking cessation clinics in the workplace are another attractive approach, especially for employers and employees who are interested in a "smoke-free" working environment. By establishing smoke-free areas, hospitals help to stimulate this process; they can also provide clinics for educational programs. Smokenders, a private organization, uses a structured educational program and positive reinforcement. In Smokenders, there are nine weekly meetings. They involve the patients with print and film information, group counseling and a host of behavior modification techniques.

Hypnosis is a smoking cessation technique that has mixed results. For some patients, it can be very effective. Ease of hypnosis appears to be an important factor in the success rate, as well as very supportive therapists and well-motivated clients.

Fighting the addictive properties of nicotine, which are considerable, requires "stick-to-it-iveness." The cravings will usually subside in several days, and weight gain can be avoided. To repeat, the highest quitting rates require a multidisciplinary approach with emphasis on education, along with a specific program.

In summary, smoking is thought to be one of the most (if not *the* most) important risk factor in cardiovascular disease. That's the bad news. The good news is that one can stop smoking and the results of stopping can be dramatic. As we have seen, the incidence of heart attacks and sudden death goes down and the risk of developing lung disease is also reduced.

One of the most successful methods of quitting smoking is the eight-step technique suggested by the American Cancer Society and mentioned earlier in this section. We cite it more fully for those interested, those who *really* want to stop smoking—for it is these persons who have the best chance of succeeding.

1. List your reasons for and against smoking. When you come to the one, "it tastes good," sit up first thing in the morning and smell your breath. Ugh. If that's not proof enough of a disgusting habit, light up a cigarette and smell it again.

2. Change to a low-tar, low-nicotine cigarette (if you don't already smoke them) and select a Q (quit) Day. This is usually a month away.

3. Chart your smoking habits for at least two weeks. Write down how many cigarettes you smoke and when you smoke them. (We suggest that you note *where* you smoke them, as well.) Many people, for example, smoke extensively on the phone (especially when speaking with an anxiety-producing friend or relative) or in the kitchen. Go over this list and rank which cigarette you think is the most important or desirable to you, such as the one with the morning coffee or the one at your desk; the next most important one; and so on down to the least important.

4. Eliminate one of the cigarettes you routinely smoke. It may be the most important one, one in the middle of your list, or the least important one.

5. Secure a supply of "oral substitutes:" mints, gum, ginger root or mouthwash, and use it instead of reaching for a cigarette (carrots and celery are also good).

6. Each night repeat at least 10 times one of your reasons for not smoking, such as having clean-smelling clothes and hair.

7. Quit on Q Day (not a day after or a day before). Try different substitutes as the urge to smoke returns. Enlist your friends or spouse in a series of busy events, such as movies, theater, a game of tennis or a walk in the fresh air.

8. Keep reminding yourself, again and again, of the four main and frightening risks of cigarette smoking—strokes, heart disease, cancer, emphysema.

Personal Views on Smoking

People often have questions related to the cessation of smoking. Since one of us (JKC) was a smoker who quit 10 years ago, she offers some personal helpful hints:

1. Do the number and kinds of cigarettes make a difference? It's better to smoke low-tar and nicotine cigarettes, but your risk is still at least 50% higher than the non-smoker. Before I quit entirely, I "cut down" to 10 cigarettes per day.

I proudly announced this fact, which I found rather formidable, to a leading heart surgeon at a social gathering. He turned to me and asked if I was really sure my breathing capacity was adequate at that level—perhaps I ought to cut down to three cigarettes a day!

2. Is any "stop-smoking" method better than another? Some people get a great deal of strength and resolve from being part of a supportive group network. Others like to do it alone or use hypnotherapy. Most of the people who have stopped smoking have done it alone; however, this may not be best for you. Methods may range from no charge to costing hundreds of dollars. Some people feel if they pay, they will stop.

3. Does everyone gain weight when they stop smoking? NO. I didn't, and one doesn't have to. However, it is a time that seems particularly easy to eat so one must be careful. Some helpful hints are:

a. Drink lots of water—at least eight glasses a day. Water is good for you; it helps to flush the poisons from the cigarettes out of your system and also helps to decrease your hunger.

b. When you drink other fluids besides water, avoid caffeine. It may make you jittery and trigger a desire for a cigarette. Some people feel a decrease in energy between 3:00 and 5:00 p.m. and are used to having a sweet or a cigarette (perhaps a reason for the English teatime). Instead, drink a glass of orange juice and, if possible, do something physical—take a walk or go for a bike ride—to minimize that low feeling.

c. Keep cut-up veggies in the refrigerator so that if you're tempted to eat, you don't reach for a high-calorie snack.

d. If you normally would talk to your aunt, who makes you quite nervous, on the phone in the kitchen while having a cigarette, talk to her somewhere else in the house. That way the cigarette won't be replaced by food.

e. Try to get some physical exercise. Breathe in clean, fresh air like you couldn't before. Exercise also gives you more energy, strange as it sounds! I started jogging and found it to be a relaxing, fun way to help maintain ideal body weight and muscle.

4. What advice should we give children? Our older son saw me writing this section on smoking and reminded me to include some words about the problem of adolescent smoking. We were living in Europe at the time, and all his friends over the age of 15 were smokers. He asked me why. I replied that children mimic the ways of their parents and then their peers. In Europe, a large percentage of the adult population continues to smoke, while they give lip service to the hazards of cigarettes.

Children learn what they see. If indeed you smoke, stop for your health, as well as that of your children. "Do as I say, not as I do" is never a satisfactory way for children to learn. They receive a mixed message. Mother or father does things one way, but I must do them another. "Which way is the right way?" they wonder. The best way for children to learn anything is by role modeling (copying the behavior of an adult the child admires).

One of the most far-reaching clinical trials that tried to control cigarette smoking and other risk factors was the Multiple Risk Factor Intervention Trial. This had the very apt acronym of MRFIT. In this study, men were motivated to not only stop smoking but also reduce their cholesterol level and their blood pressure. Two groups were involved: One received the "usual" care from their own physicians, and the other received more intensive care from a specialized protocol. At the end of the study period, a 1982 report showed the expected number of deaths from coronary artery disease was decreased in both groups, indicating that even usual care in today's health-conscious world can result in lowered cholesterol levels, blood pressure and cigarette usage.

Control of high blood pressure can be simple for many of the nearly 60 million people with this problem in the United States. Reducing salt, losing weight and a good exercise program can do wonders. Low-sodium diets are discussed in the following chapter. When these measures are not enough to lower the blood pressure to normal levels, there are a variety of medications that can be taken once or twice a day (with few side effects). Surgery on the kidneys and/or its blood vessels is no longer considered as effective therapy for any but a very small number (2%) of hypertensive patients. Except for these rare cases, it is not necessary. Drugs to treat high blood pressure fall into one of three categories: diuretics, vasodilators and nervous system inhibitors.

Diuretics (water pills) cause the body to excrete salt (sodium) and water. This reduces excess fluid in the body and, more importantly, relieves the tension in the blood vessel wall that is caused by salt retention. As a result, the body has a diuresis (excretion of fluid), and urine flow increases. It is surprising how many individuals see their blood pressure fall to a normal range with only the addition of a once-a-day water pill. Types of diuretic pills include those with and those without potassium- and magnesium-retaining abilities. We consider this an important consideration for the following reason: Many cardiologists feel strongly that low levels of potassium and magnesium in the blood (from diuretics) can contribute to the development of fatal heart irregularities (arrhythmias) in patients with underlying heart disease. Low levels in these persons could be harmless—or disastrous. Physicians who are not cardiologists appear less concerned because most of their patients on diuretics do not have these problems. True, the odds are that it will cause no harm, but cardiologists see enough patients with arrhythmias in coronary care units who have low levels as a result of diuretic therapy to be concerned about this problem. Thus, we recommend using only those diuretics with potassium- and preferably also magnesium-retaining abilities. Some doctors recommend potassium supplements instead. Discuss this with your doctor if a diuretic is prescribed for you.

The second type of medication, vasodilators (blood vessel expanders), act by relaxing the muscles in the wall of the arteries throughout the body that control the level of blood pressure. Some of these drugs (such as the calcium blockers) are also used to treat episodes of ischemia (see Chapter 10). Other drugs are captopril (Capoten), enalapril (Vasotec), lisinopril (Zestril), ramipril (Altace) and quinapril (Accupril), all angiotension-converting-enzyme inhibitors that help lower blood pressure.

The drugs that interfere with central nervous system impulses can do so in a variety of ways. The beta blockers interfere with the action of the "active" chemical that comes from nerve endings. They are also used to treat ischemia and are discussed at length in Chapter 10. Other drugs act on the brain to control the flow of impulses. These include methyldopa (trade name Aldomet), clonidine (Catapres), prazosin (Minipress), and the newest doxazosin (Cardura).

All drugs have side effects. Use of any of them should be thoroughly discussed with your doctor. How does he or she decide with which drugs to start? This depends on your age, race and level of activity. Experience has shown, for example, that people under the age of 40 respond better to beta blockers than do older people in whom a diuretic is usually the first choice. After the initial medication, drugs with different actions are added in a step-wise manner until blood pressure is controlled. The goal is to achieve a reasonable blood pressure (lower than 140/90) without undesirable side effects. When high blood pressure is treated successfully, the long-term results speak for themselves. Effective control means reduced mortality and fewer deaths due to stroke, heart failure or kidney disease. Clinical trials in the United States, Australia and Sweden clearly show this benefit when the diastolic blood pressure is initially above 105 mm mercury. In the late 1970s, milder degrees of high blood pressure (diastolics between 90 and 105 mm) were examined in the Hypertension Detection and Follow-up Program in the United States and in the Australian Therapeutic Trial and showed similar results, though these have been challenged by some. We side with those who advocate treatment of *all* hypertension with the caveat that drug regimens must be carefully monitored. Unfortunately, none of the studies show a statistically significant decline in heart attacks, though the trend is there.

In conclusion, control of high cholesterol levels, stopping cigarette smoking and reduction of high blood pressure are "do-able." With such control will come a reduction in risk of developing heart disease! What better impetus to healthy living habits does one need?

CHAPTER

8

How to Eat
a Heart-Healthy Diet
and Still Enjoy Yourself

Healthy and moderate eating habits need to be a way of life for all Americans. One can modulate eating habits at home and in restaurants and still eat without feeling deprived. Favorite meals can be adapted to your diet, and new and exciting recipes can find a place in your kitchen. To help you, a week of heart-healthy—and delicious—dinner menus are provided at the end of this book. For those with significant blood cholesterol problems, specific drug programs are suggested.

High blood cholesterol levels and, to a lesser extent, obesity are risk factors for coronary artery disease. Can a person eat well and still enjoy meals? We think so, and the goal of this chapter is to give practical suggestions on how to do it.

The heart and lungs have to work excessively hard when a person is obese. Twenty-five percent of problems associated with heart disease are related to a person being overweight. Obesity is a major contributing cause of high blood pressure; hypertension is twice as common in obese people as in slender people.

Weight loss can bring down blood pressure as well as high cholesterol levels. Not only are obesity and poor eating habits associated with heart disease, they are also associated with diabetes, strokes, and, according to researchers, some cancers.

In a 1992 article in The New England Journal of Medicine, researchers from St. Luke's Hospital in New York City reported that obese people overestimate their physical activities and underestimate the amount of food they eat. They also report that many obese people attribute their condition to thyroid problems, but in reality, the reason they are heavy is because of their nutritional habits.

Often, one will hear thin people accused of always being on a diet. We don't believe that crash dieting is the answer to weight control, nor do most other people concerned with good nutrition. To be effective, healthy eating habits need to become a way of life. Many people who have successfully overcome their weight problem find that they just don't eat as much as they once did even after they think their "dieting period" is over. One can thus conclude that a fit person "lives" a healthy diet.

When should healthy eating habits begin? When should fat-rich foods be minimized? Some believe that it should start at birth, though there is still controversy about this and many pediatricians suggest waiting until infancy is over. The American Heart Association suggests waiting until age two before such foods are reduced.

In this chapter on nutrition, much of the information is devoted to developing a daily way of life: a new lifestyle. Those people who have already been diagnosed with cardiovascular disease will have to take special precautions to eat food that is *both low in fat and in calories*. Once again, remember that moderation is the key; good, healthful eating does not mean that your favorite food—whatever it may be—needs to be deleted from your plate forever.

When we were young, our parents felt inadequate unless they provided us with meat, two starches, vegetable, salad and homemade dessert at dinner. Thank goodness, times have changed, and we have come to realize that overeating starts in childhood and can only be harmful to one's health. Unfortunately, food is used with children both as punishment and as a reward. Children often equate mother's loving feelings (or lack of them) with food. Thus, people often overeat because they are being rewarded or are substituting food for mother's affection. Most children (as most adults) have a built-in mechanism that indicates when they are full and thus have no more need to eat. If we teach ourselves (and our children) to listen to and heed the advice given by this device, no one need be obese. (The prevalence of genetic obesity remains to be determined.) Try to eat only when you are hungry and only until you are full.

Many of our patients need to control their weight. Here are some of the suggestions we give to them that may be helpful to you:

1. Make a list of when and where you eat. Do you taste a bite of everything when you prepare dinner and then eat again as if you hadn't eaten since lunch? Do you eat peanuts, crackers, or ice cream incessantly while watching TV or reading? Do you finish the pint of ice cream that was half full while you talk on the telephone in the kitchen? Do you eat when you are depressed, tense, anxious, or particularly pleased with your accomplishments? Be aware if you eat because of your emotional state.

2. Eat only when hungry and only until full—if you are particularly hungry, try to eat something small and wait 20 minutes before consuming more food. The brain does not get a message of fullness from the stomach until after a delay.

3. Try to eat only when you are sitting down, and don't participate in any other activity while you are eating. You will become more aware of the texture, smell, and taste of whatever you eat so that you get more satisfaction from it, perhaps eating less of it. On the other hand, if you find that you are full or that what you are eating is distasteful, you are less likely to finish the portion when you are totally aware of what you are consuming.

Here are some other handy hints for changing habits of eating fattening food:

1. Buy or make cookies or cakes that you won't eat. For example, our children like cookies and cakes without nuts; we love them with nuts. Thus, all cookies, except maybe one or two in a batch, will be made without nuts! If you buy cookies, buy those the children like and you can do without.

2. Try to make your cupboards and refrigerator temptation proof. If you have leftover puddings and pies from a holiday meal, put them in the back of the refrigerator while the veggies occupy the proud position in front. If your house just has to have junk food, put it in the back of the cupboard. When fattening food is less accessible, one has to think about whether one really should indulge.

3. Eat slowly. Not only is eating more enjoyable and polite in this manner, but one is less likely to eat two or three portions while one's family or friends are only eating one. Also remember that it takes time for the brain to get the message from the stomach that it is full, so wait a while before taking another serving.

4. Spend less time in the kitchen. In the last 20 years, houses in the United States seem to be constructed with large kitchens and/or adjoining family rooms. That way, everyone has access to the kitchen at all times. It's better to prepare the food, eat it, clean it up and be out of the kitchen. There's less temptation, and you have to really be conscious of wanting to eat if you have to walk from another room in the house.

5. Go grocery shopping when you are not hungry, prepared with a list indicating the foods that you need. Hunger in a market translates into reckless buying of fattening food, often consumed in the market or on the way home.

6. Try to have someone in the family without a weight problem put away the leftovers. Frequently people eat the remainder of the rice, noodles, or dessert while they are cleaning up because there is not really enough for an additional meal.

7. Eat one small serving of food and don't serve it on a gigantic plate. When one is eating small quantities of food, a

large plate exaggerates the small portions and increases the feelings of deprivation.

8. Certain times of the day precipitate nibbling or snacking. Often it is right before dinner. If possible, try to get some exercise at that time by taking a walk or going for a bike ride. If that's not possible, put healthful, low-fattening snack food (e.g., cut-up celery, lettuce, carrots, zucchini) in the front of your refrigerator for munching.

9. Change your cooking habits.

    a. The new cooking pans such as "T-Fal" or "Silver-stone" are excellent and need no oil or margarine for frying. Stir-frying can be done with water instead of oil when using these pans. Remember, each table-spoon of fat, whether it be oil, butter, or margarine, contains 100 calories!

    b. Revise your favorite recipes. For example, most reci-pes call for an excessive amount of sugar and fat. We usually reduce the amount by at least a half, taste and then use more if necessary.

The American Heart Association suggests putting your favorite recipes "on a diet." In order to cut back on the fats (butter, margarine, and oils) one must substitute other fluids, such as chicken stock or vegetable broth. When making casseroles, cut down on the meat by using more vegetables, beans, and grains. Or, how about using ground chicken or turkey meat instead of beef in casseroles, meat loaf, or spa-ghetti sauce? Since one usually uses strong spices in these meals, the taste is not changed dramatically. When making Oriental food such as moo-shi pork, substitute chicken or turkey for the meat. When you bake, there are many substi-tutes that one can make for the high fat and caloric ingredi-ents such as butter, sour cream, eggs, and whole milk. Egg whites can often be substituted for whole eggs; butter can always be replaced by margarine, buttermilk, water; prune puree or applesauce can often be used to replace fats in baking. Recently, I made a pumpkin bread that called for one cup oil and one cup orange juice. I replaced 3/4 cup of the oil with additional orange juice. The bread produced was more moist, tastier, less fatty, and less greasy. However, in many recipes, one cannot eliminate all fat or the results will be dry and tasteless. Most importantly, don't tell the family that the new or revised recipe is good for them. You might unnecessarily cause a revolution in the ranks.

WHAT IS A "PROPER" DIET?

By this time it has become obvious that cholesterol is one of the main culprits in the heart disease epidemic. For a small number of individuals, the cause of their high blood cholesterol levels is due purely and simply to a genetic fault. Because of this genetic fault, the LDL receptor in liver cells is either partially or totally defective from birth. Cholesterol cannot be cleared normally from the blood. Heart attacks do occur in young people, even children. Fortunately, only a small percentage of all heart attacks are due to this condition. Work in elucidating this defective gene won the 1985 Nobel Prize in medicine and physiology for Drs. Michael Brown and Joseph Goldstein of the University of Texas Health Science Center in Dallas.

At the present time, our only explanation for the high cholesterol levels in most heart attack victims involves environmental rather than genetic factors. Such people ingest too much cholesterol and too much saturated fat which is converted to cholesterol by the body. Therefore, the goal of proper eating habits is to reduce the consumption of cholesterol and fats, especially animal (saturated) fats so that the blood cholesterol level is lower than 240 mg% and as close to 200 mg% as possible. Under 200 mg% is optimum. The average American's fat intake is around 40% of total calories. This is too high. In 1986, the American Heart Association revised its recommendation for a proper diet. It now recommends no more than 30% fats with 10% or less coming from animal fats. Cholesterol intake should not exceed 300mg per day. The recommendations in this chapter are based on those recommended not only by the American Heart Association but by the 1991 report of the Expert Panel on Population Strategies for Blood Cholesterol Reduction (a federally funded project). The experts say (and so do we) that one has to be leary of food and diet fads. We know that whole grains are fat free, healthful and aid in digestion. However, they are not panaceas for everything and anything. For example, about three years ago, oat bran was touted as being the cure for high levels of cholesterol. Although adding oat bran to foods, eating it as breakfast cereal by itself or combined with oatmeal may be tasty and healthful, it has not been proven that it has any additional benefits in controlling cholesterol levels compared to other grains.

Types of Fats
Saturated (ideally to be avoided because they increase the cholesterol in your blood):

Pistachio nuts
Macadamia nuts
Palm and coconut oil
Butter
Cheese
Meat
Homogenized milk
Chocolate chips and unsweetened chocolate
Cream
Egg Yolk
Ice Cream

Monosaturated (to be used in moderation because they don't effect the cholesterol one way or the other):

Avocado
Cashew nuts
Olive oil
Peanuts

Polyunsaturated (can be used more frequently because they lower the amount of cholesterol in the blood):

Walnuts
Safflower oil
Fish
Sunflower oil
Corn oil
Almonds
Corn and safflower oil margarine
Pecans

The recommendation for lowering animal fats in the diet reflects the fact that some societies (Eskimos, Japanese, and some Mediterranean peoples) eat a lot of fat, but have little coronary artery disease. The reason? They have a very low intake of *saturated fats*. Most of the fat in Mediterranean diets comes from slightly saturated vegetable fats, such as olive oil. The low coronary death rates in Eskimos and Japanese people have been attributed to their fish consumption. The polyunsaturated fatty acids in fish oil (the "omega-3" family) seem to be responsible. Not only do they belong to the class of fats associated with low blood cholesterol (the polyunsaturates), but they also possess anti-platelet effects. Remembering how key the platelet is to clot formation in coronary arteries (Chapter 4), we now understand why studies in 1985 and 1986 linking fish oils to reduced coronary blockages in humans and experimental animals received so much interest. One study from the Netherlands suggested that the consumption of as few as one or two fish dishes per week may be of value in preventing heart attacks! Because of uncertainties about the side effects of capsules containing omega-3 rich fish oil supplements, we recommend you eat the fish and avoid the capsules until more is known about them. Additional evidence of the importance of a healthy diet comes from the fact that vegetarians have the lowest rates of coronary artery disease in the world! Their diet is virtually devoid of all saturated fats. Based on what we have written above, we feel it is unnecessary to go to extremes of any kind in order to eat and live "heart healthy," but we do recommend less meat, more fish, skinned poultry, vegetables, and grains.

One of the most important ideas about food doses came out of the U.S. Department of Agriculture recently. This is the concept of the Food Pyramid. What it means is that food consumption should consist mainly of bread, rice, cereal, and pasta (the base of the pyramid), followed by vegetables, dairy, meat, fish, eggs, and nuts. One should use fats, oils, and sweets as little as possible (the top of the pyramid).

If diet doesn't work, there are also drugs available for low-ering blood cholesterol levels. The oldest of these are called *bile acid sequestering resins*—a bit of a tongue twister! Very simply, these oral agents form a non-digestible complex with cholesterol in the bowel and cause it to be excreted in the stool. Choles-tyramine (brand name Questran) is the most popular of these agents. It can have undesirable gastrointestinal side effects, and should be used only by persons with elevated cholesterol levels whose attempts at dietary lowering of cholesterol have been unsuccessful. Other drugs are also available, such as colestipol (brand name Colestid), probucol (Lorelco), gemfibrozil (Lopid), and an old standby, niacin. The most promising of the newer drugs, which block the production of cholesterol by the liver are lovastatin (Mevacor), the most widely used, pravastatin (Prava-chol), and zimvastatin (Zocor). These drugs are used mostly in people with *known* heart disease. Anti-oxidants such as Vitamin C and especially Vitamin E (in a daily dose of 400 international units) can reduce the harmful effects of cholesterol by a different mechanism. Anti-oxidants represent an exciting innovation in this field, and we suspect much more will be written about them.

Three other food ingredients—salt, alcohol, and caffeine—warrant comment. For persons with high blood pressure or fluid buildup, one should eliminate salt. If one cannot lower one's blood pressure or fluid buildup by these measures, one should take diuretics (which increase salt and fluid loss) under a doctor's direction.

Salt is bad for us, as noted earlier, but most of us continue to use it in excess quantities. It is an acquired taste: babies look disgusted when given something salty to taste, and yet teenagers seem to eat anything and everything that contains salt. Current guidelines suggest consuming a maximum of one teaspoon (3g) of salt per day. How can a family begin to decrease their consumption of salt to more acceptable levels?

1. Avoid fast food restaurants.
2. Avoid processed food (especially meats), TV dinners, canned soups.
3. Use unsalted margarine.
4. Taste all food before considering the use of salt. We are always confounded by people who add salt without knowing whether the cook has added it.
5. Avoid putting a salt shaker on the table. To use your favorite recipes but reduce consumption of salt, try adding half the salt recommended. Next time cut it in half again until such time that you use a sprinkle or none at all.
6. Try using herbs and spices instead of salt. Garlic, onions, mustard, and lemons are very tasty common ingredients found in most households. If you like, try all the herbs and spices you can find. Tex-Mex and Cajun cooking require no salt because of the strong spicy flavors. They often make food more interesting and definitely make it more healthful.
7. Instead of salt, use sherry or wine to flavor soups, stews, and sauces. By cooking for at least 30 minutes, the alcohol evaporates, but the flavor remains.
8. Add additional amounts of extracts (vanilla, chocolate, coconut, almond butter, etc.) to cakes and pies for flavor instead of salt.
9. The American Heart Association often gives away a cookbook with a donation, such as *Cooking Without Salt*, which will give you many suggestions for a new way of cooking while also benefiting research projects on heart disease. There are many other such books on the bookstore shelves.

The following is a list of foods that are high in sodium and should be eliminated from the diet of anyone who has high blood pressure or heart problems related to retention of fluids. For others, *these are the foods to be avoided or used in moderation:*

anchovies and anchovy paste
bacon
baked beans with pork
baking powder
beef, corned and dried
bouillon cubes (except low
    sodium; check label)
canned vegetables
crab, canned
crackers, soda type
catsup in large quantities
celery salt
cereals (check label; the best
    ones will have less than
    250 mg per serving)
cheese (blue, cheddar, pro-
    cessed; use in moderation)

corn, popped with salt added
fish, smoked
meats, smoked
olives
peanuts, salted
pickles
potato chips and other simi-
    larly salted snack foods
pretzels, salted
processed luncheon meats
salad dressings
sauerkraut
sausage, frankfurters
soups, canned
soy sauce
TV dinners (check labels)
Worchestershire sauce

The following foods have a natural diuretic function and help your body get rid of salt and water:

apricots
asparagus
bananas
broccoli
cantaloupe
chicken
cottage cheese
figs
grapefruit and grapefruit juice
milk, skim and low-fat

nuts, unsalted
oranges and orange juice
pineapple, fresh
potatoes
prunes and prune juice
raisins
tomatoes
tuna, water packed
turkey
watermelon

Alcohol is another problem. There is no evidence that it causes coronary artery disease, and, in fact, there is some evidence that coronary artery disease occurs less in people who drink *moderately* (one drink per day). Three drinks or more can cause cardiovascular problems, though not heart attacks. Does red wine really protect the French foie-gras eaters from heart attacks? Despite the hoopla, there is no solid evidence to back up such claims.

There is some evidence that caffeine can cause or aggravate arrhythmias (heart beat irregularities). Therefore, in persons with a history of arrhythmias, decaffeinated beverages are recommended. Since coffee, tea, and soft drinks all come in decaffeinated forms, this should prove no problem to the concerned consumer. We do not feel that there is conclusive evidence indicating that substances used to decaffeinate coffee and tea contain carcinogens. Whether or not drinking coffee can also contribute to plaque formation in the coronary arteries (that is, whether it is a true risk factor) is unclear. In the Framingham Study, people who smoked and drank excessive amounts of coffee had a higher level of cardiac mortality. A 1986 report by Dr. Andrea LaCroix and colleagues at Johns Hopkins found an independent link between coffee intake and coronary artery disease. Those who drank five or more cups per day had a two to three times greater in risk of developing cardiac events compared to nondrinkers. When the subject was reviewed more recently in a 1992 report in the Archives of Internal Medicine, this conclusion could not be confirmed, but moderation seems a good recommendation.

HOW TO BE A SUPER SUPERMARKET SHOPPER

Shopping can often cause problems for people who would like to eat less as well as consume healthful foods. Never shop when you are hungry. Research has shown that people are more apt to buy more food at that time. One will also tend to purchase food that does not accede to a dietary or monetary budget. In other words, one is often frivolous when marketing while hungry.

In order to plan interesting and varied menus for the week, make a list before you go shopping and purchase only those items on the list. This helps organize the life of the busy family, while cutting down on excessive buying and trips to the market. Varied and interesting menus help people feel less deprived when they are trying to maintain or lose weight. One week can include seafood, veal, chicken, pasta, vegetarian meals, Oriental dishes, fish, and beef. If you take a weekend day to cook and freeze, you can pop the frozen meal in the oven or microwave, thereby avoiding weekday preparation time and the use of commercially made food that is expensive and often unhealthful.

Use fresh fruits and vegetables. They are more tasty and often less expensive than the canned or frozen types. Instead of smothering vegetables with margarine, try steaming them until crunchy and eating them plain or with a sprinkle of herbs. Vegetables have wonderful flavors of their own that are frequently obscured by sauces. Fresh fruits are a delicious snack or dessert that satisfy the desire for sweets.

It is important to read labels while shopping, especially if you eat already prepared food. New legislation requires that most foods list amounts of sodium, fat, sugar, cholesterol, and calories. However, at present, the way in which the law was written makes it difficult for people to compare similar products. More consistent labeling will be seen in the future which will make managing a heart-healthy diet easier.

If you do have to resort to TV dinners, be sure to read the label so that you are aware of the following things before you purchase them:

1. How many calories are in one serving?
2. How much fat is in one serving—make sure that there are under 10g per 300 calories.
3. How much sodium or salt is in one service: if noted, make sure there is not more than 1000mg. If salt is not mentioned, but words containing "sodium" are mentioned, more times than not it is probably too salty and should not be purchased.
4. Compare two brands of the same product. Select the one that has less salt and fat.

When choosing bread products, remember that pita bread, rice cakes, and unfried tortillas contain little or no fat. Italian, French, whole-grain, and partially whole-grain bread are low-fat items. English muffins, sandwich rolls, and water bagels also contain little fat. Many new bread products are being marketed with little or no fat, but the cereal aisle is still filled with cereals that contain huge amounts of fats, sugar, and salt. Try buying cereal that has not already been sweetened. Pre-sweetened cereals contain so much sugar that the predominant ingredients are sugar or corn syrup (another kind of sugar). Buy hot cereals that are not labelled "instant." When cooking these cereals oneself, one need not add salt—an ingredient often excessively used in the instant varieties. Most granola cereals that are not prepared at home contain coconut or palm oil, brown sugar, salt, cane sugar, and honey, and thus are fattening and unhealthful. Although the oats, seeds, nuts, and fruits are healthful, when combined with the other ingredients the cereal becomes fattening and unhealthful because of the sugars, and full of cholesterol because of the palm and coconut oil.

By planning one's shopping, one can become a super supermarket shopper who saves cholesterol, salt, calories, and money!

RESTAURANT EATING: MAINTAINING OR LOSING WEIGHT

Many busy men and women choose to, or have to, eat many of their meals at restaurants. Often we are asked how one can lose or maintain one's weight when eating out. Here are some suggestions:

1. One doesn't have to eat everything on one's plate. We often find that restaurants give you too much food. Divide your portion in half, wait a few minutes, and see if you really want the rest; in other words, are you still hungry? If you are not, ask for a doggie bag or give it to a friend.
2. Don't order a set menu with four, five, or six courses—order à la carte. We have found that even though one may have the right intentions, one might feel compelled to at least taste each course. At the end of a large set menu, one is far more likely to feel sick than satisfied because of the excess food consumed.

3. Taste the food—if you don't like it, are full, or have another course coming, don't eat it, but have it taken away by the waiter. If it remains, you may nibble at it.

4. To avoid fats that are unhealthy and fattening, avoid food made with cream (soups, quiche, cream sauces). We have started to inquire before ordering whether sauces contain cream. Once one avoids cream for a while, it no longer tastes good.

5. Ask for any sauces, gravies and dressings to be served in a separate dish. Avoid using them altogether or use them sparingly, knowing that most sauces contain a great deal of oil and salt.

6. Ask that vegetables be served without butter or margarine. Often restaurants put so much butter on their vegetables that they don't taste good and are also very fattening.

7. Try to avoid fattening desserts. Either order fruit, share a portion with a friend or just have a bite. If you have a "sweet tooth," having just a little can be as satisfying as finishing the entire dessert.

8. A new "style" or "way" of eating is to order two appetizers and a salad (or just one appetizer and a salad) if you're watching your calorie intake or don't want too much food. Appetizers are often the most interesting part of the menu and are often quite large.

9. Do not worry about the *occasional* splurge. Don't deprive yourself on your birthday! Just get back to eating normally the next day.

10. Perhaps the most important thing about eating in restaurants or eating in general is *moderation*.

CHAPTER
9

To Exercise
or Not to Exercise?

Studies from around the world show the same trend: Physically inactive people are at greater risk of developing heart disease than are active people. If an exercise program is to be followed—and we strongly believe in the merits of such a program—the best kind of exercise is one that uses the large muscles of the body in a steady contraction–relaxation pattern (running, walking, swimming, biking). All people over the age of 35—especially men—who are about to begin physical fitness programs and have risk factors for heart disease should first consult with their doctor about having an exercise electrocardiogram performed to detect silent heart disease.

Outside the window of the room in London where this chapter is being written, two seemingly unrelated events are occurring. A red double-decker bus—one of the sights that identifies London to the rest of the world—is slowly chugging down Sloane Street. Behind it on the sidewalk a jogger, clad in shorts and a sleeveless running shirt, is moving quickly down the street. Soon the jogger overtakes the bus and disappears, paying no more attention to the bus than he would a tree! What the runner doesn't know—and what most people don't know—is that the bus (or more properly, the people who work on it) is one of the reasons there is a jogging craze in the United States and the beginning of similar trends all over the Western world. What is the relation between London bus workers and joggers? Read on!

It is no secret that most Americans—even young ones—are not physically fit. The President's Council on Physical Fitness reported distressing statistics on the subject in reference to school-age children. The Amateur Athletic Union found that this disappointing trend intensified, rather than improved, as children got older: High school students were less physically fit than junior high school students! It is not surprising that the situation in adults is equally sobering. In 1982, a survey of lifestyles of Massachusetts residents was published. Among the findings: Almost 30% did not exercise at all; only 10% exercised more than 1 hour per day.

It is true that some decline in activity is "normal" as people age. Thus, the ability to raise the heart rate, which is the single most important aspect of cardiovascular fitness, normally diminishes with age. This often can be compensated for by a proper conditioning program. Most of the decline in cardiovascular fitness is due to a lack of conditioning: If you don't use a muscle frequently (any muscle) it grows flabby. The scientific term for this is "disuse atrophy." If you couple disuse atrophy with weight gain—a common phenomenon in our society where we add pounds as we add years—you have less efficient muscles. A muscular structure like the heart now has to work extra hard just to maintain its normal output.

All right, the reader will concede, I accept all these things. But I don't like to exercise and I don't want to exercise, so why should I? Where is the evidence that it does me any good—like protecting me against heart attacks? I've heard lots of stuff lately about it all being a myth anyway.

Fair enough. In this chapter, we will present the evidence, pro and con. But we want to warn the reader before we begin:

We are biased, since we both excise regularly, jogging about 20–30 miles per week. Obviously, we are not doing this just to keep the domestic running shoe industry in business! We believe in the benefits of exercise, but we will present the facts as they are and let the readers form their own opinions.

THE PROS

The beginning of the "exercise hypothesis" can be said to date, indirectly, from the 1950s, when a number of intriguing statistics on occupational mortality in Great Britain were released. Because these reports found that deaths from heart disease were more common in white-collar workers than in blue-collar workers, they suggested that people in sedentary occupations were more prone to heart attacks than those in more active occupations. To follow up on this assumption, Dr. J. N. Morris and colleagues published a landmark study in 1953. These investigators studied the mortality statistics of over 30,000 London bus drivers as compared to those of the conductors. In the British system, the bus drivers do not collect the fare—they merely drive the buses. It is the conductors who march up and down the aisles of the double decker buses collecting the fares. The former is clearly a sedentary occupation, the latter is not. Dr. Morris found that, as a group, the drivers had twice the rate of heart disease (heart attacks and death) as did the conductors. Furthermore, drivers under 50 years of age had three times as many sudden deaths as a similar age group of conductors.

One must be careful in studies like this to make sure there are not confounding factors; that is, a greater prevalence of coronary risk factors present in the drivers. As it turned out, when Dr. Morris and colleagues re-studied the two groups (because they too were aware of the limitations of their study), there *were* higher levels of both cholesterol and blood pressure in the drivers. This deflated somewhat the conclusions emphasizing the importance of physical activity, since it could very well be that bus driver recruits started out with a worse coronary risk profile. One could argue that these individuals, especially since they were also heavier, would gravitate toward less physically demanding jobs. The other variable that had to be examined was the level of leisure time activity in the two groups. What if drivers were more active in their off hours than conductors? This would also negate the effect of their work habits. To pursue this latter point, Dr. Morris performed a subsequent study (published in 1973) involving nearly 18,000 British civil servants, all of whom had similar types of desk jobs. Those civil servants who were more physically active in their leisure time (sports, housework, gardening) had fewer heart attacks. Again, there was no attempt to match the presence of coronary risk factors, but the trend persisted, even in subgroups with many risk factors and subgroups with few risk factors.

Despite these impressive results, there are those who argue against the conclusive nature of the findings. They use the convenient argument of self-selection. Again and again we will hear critics say those who exercise are more resistant (in some unknown fashion) to heart disease in the first place and that whatever they do in regard to work activities or physical fitness in their leisure hours doesn't really matter. This is a nihilistic approach. Common sense, as Dr. Morris himself noted in defense of his studies, would suggest that although different types of men choose different types of jobs, their exercise habits in the next 20–40 years should also influence their health.

What are the other studies that back up Dr. Morris's premise? And what are the studies that refute it? In support of Dr. Morris's data are general population studies from Framingham, Massachusetts (this is the Framingham Study, referred to throughout this book), as well as those from Georgia, Iowa, Puerto Rico and Israel. The Framingham Study showed that sedentary men were at greater risk of developing heart disease *no matter what the level of conventional risk factors*. The Georgia and Iowa studies looked at farmers versus non-farmers. The Iowa data are particularly interesting. We think of a farm diet as being rich in eggs and other dairy products and red meat—which in many cases it is. This should translate into higher levels of blood cholesterol—which it often does. Despite this, the Iowa farmers had a lower incidence of heart disease than the statewide average for all men. This prompted a 1982 report comparing the physical fitness of a group of farmers and non-farmers. The farmers proved to be more physically fit. The treadmill exercise test showed they had lower resting heart rates (a sign of fitness) and could exercise longer on the treadmill before becoming fatigued. They also smoked less. Conclusion: if you're active—and a non-smoker—a farmer's diet is not as bad as it may seem. The Georgia report followed farmers and non-farmers for seven years after introduction into the study, with the same conclusions as in Iowa. The Puerto Rican comparison of rural and urban men also showed that the rural men—who were more physically active—had a lower incidence of heart disease. They also tended to have lower levels of coronary risk factors.

Wait a minute, say the skeptics, here we go again! Which comes first, the chicken or the egg? But does it matter? Perhaps they go together—perhaps exercise reduces serum cholesterol levels and blood pressure. And it is extremely difficult to smoke a cigarette while running!

The Israeli experience dealt with workers on a kibbutz (farm cooperative). Those with sedentary jobs fared worse in regard to developing heart disease than did more active workers. Self-selection? Perhaps, but it seems to fit the pattern we have been describing.

Several studies have attempted to quantify the amount of physical activity undertaken by the study participants. Some of the best known of these have come from the work of Dr. Ralph Paffenbarger and colleagues at the Stanford University School of Medicine. In an early study, they evaluated over 3000 San Franciscan longshoremen. They divided the men into light duty and heavy duty workers, based on the amount of calories expended per day. Sudden deaths from heart disease were three times greater in the light-duty workers. After adjusting the two groups for differences in the conventional risk factors (plus other factors such as race, history of heart disease, etc.) they still found that the heavy duty workers had a much lower frequency of fatal heart attacks. The investigators wanted to make certain that other variables were not confounding these results. So thorough were they that they even took into account people who started out in light duty jobs and then were transferred from light to heavy duty and vice versa, before the fatal event!

Perhaps the most famous of Dr. Paffenbarger's studies are those involving almost 17,000 Harvard College alumni. A physical fitness index was devised to assess the level of their activity. Data were obtained by questionnaires and college records. About half the group expended under 2000 calories* a week in "extra" energy (stair climbing, walking, sports), and half the group expended more than 2000 calories per week. In the initial report dealing with the 6–10 year follow-up period, there was a clear indication that those in the lower energy group had a higher incidence of cardiac events. In the most recent report detailing the 12–16 year follow-up period (published in 1986), the initial trend was confirmed. There was a trend toward steady reduction in death rates as the energy expended on the aforementioned activities increased from less than 500 to 3500 calories per week. Even considering the effects of conventional risk factors, plus the gain in body weight and presence of parental heart disease, "alumni mortality rates were significally lower among the physically active." (Not surprisingly, the highest death rates were found in those non-exercising individuals who also were cigarette smokers and had high blood pressure.) One of the interesting "extras" in Dr. Paffenbarger's study of Harvard alumni was his conclusions about college athletes. Only if they stayed active in later life did they maintain their lower risk state. Conversely, he reported in 1986 that non-athletes who developed an active fitness profile (expending 2000 or more calories a week on walking, sports, etc.) could become low-risk. The thoroughness of this data is in contrast to other studies of college athletes that did not consider post-college lifestyles.

---

* A calorie is a unit of energy produced by burning fuel. Burning one gram of fat releases 9 calories, while 1g of protein or carbohydrates only produces 4 calories.

These population studies do not provide direct information on how physically fit their subjects were but merely describe the amount of physical exercise or exertion they experienced in their daily lives. To assess cardiovascular fitness, one has to do what the Iowa farm study did: place the subjects on treadmills and quantify their responses. In one of the most famous of these studies, Dr. Robert Bruce and colleagues at the University of Washington tested over 4000 clinically healthy men. The presence of risk factors and development of ST depression on the exercise test adversely influenced survival over the course of the follow-up period, as did other factors including the total exercise time the person could perform. Thus, if you were not fit enough to continue on the treadmill beyond six minutes, the chance of developing a heart attack or dying was much greater. The study found that 1% of the men had a high-risk profile and that nearly a quarter of this small group had cardiac events during the 5 year follow-up period. This is truly a high-risk group, and they would be the people most suitable for more intensive evaluation. These studies dovetail nicely with the prognosis studies of Dr. Erikssen's from Norway (discussed in Chapter 5). We could argue that perhaps it is this high-risk group that should undergo the coronary arteriographic procedure described in Chapter 3.

It is not easy to weed out the importance of physical fitness from the effects of the coronary risk factors. To do this one has to show that in a randomly selected population, those who cannot exercise for long periods and who have lower maximal exercise heart rates have more heart disease during the follow-up period. This was demonstrated in a study from Sweden published in 1981. Another piece of evidence that physical fitness is important comes from the Framingham Study: The lower your resting (pre-exercise) heart rate, the less your chances of developing heart disease. Why? Lower heart rates indicate better cardiovascular conditioning (as we will discuss in more detail later in this chapter).

We believe that the evidence presented at this point makes a strong case that exercise and physical fitness help protect against heart disease. But what about those studies that show no relation between physical activity and heart disease? How numerous are they and how valid are their results?

THE CONS

The studies most commonly cited are those from Los Angeles, Chicago and Finland. The Los Angeles study involved about 1400 civil servants; the 10-year follow-up results were published in 1964. Physical activity—as estimated from job titles—did not appear to influence development of heart disease. Leisure time activity was not evaluated, nor for that matter was cigarette smoking. The Chicago study involved about 1700 workers at the Western Electric Company. The eight-year follow-up, reported in 1983, did look into both work and leisure time activity. There was a trend toward benefit from physical activity, but this trend did not reach a level of statistical significance (the mathematical end point necessary to prove a given result was not merely the result of chance). A similar trend was observed in another study when United States railroad switchmen were found to have a lower incidence of heart disease than less active railroad employees. The 1976 study from Finland actually showed a harmful effect. The group with the highest level of physical activity were lumberjacks, but they had a *higher* 10-year coronary mortality rate than did less active farmers. The lumberjacks were also heavier smokers than the farmers and they also came primarily from eastern Finland, a notoriously high coronary-prone area. Other studies of men living in this area of Finland demonstrate the expected relationship between low physical activity and high rates of heart disease in men. Why the lumberjacks are an exception is not clear. It might be that because of all the risk factors present in this area, many of the lumberjacks already have latent (silent) coronary artery disease and that vigorous physical activity places them at high risk, as we will discuss later in this chapter.

We do not believe that the data in these studies refutes the premise that physical fitness helps protect against heart disease.

EXERCISE AFTER A HEART ATTACK

Just as there are conflicting reports on whether exercise is a protective factor before heart disease develops, so too are there conflicting reports about its usefulness after a heart attack. Most towns in the United States have at least one cardiac rehabilitation center for persons recovering from heart attacks after they have been discharged from the hospital. These centers also are used for other heart patients as well, especially those recovering from open-heart surgery, but the overwhelming majority of patients are recent heart attack victims. The goal of these centers is to strengthen the heart, improve cardiovascular fitness and prevent future heart attacks. In the general sense, a rehabilitation program after any long hospitalization or illness is worthwhile since long hours spent lying in bed or sitting in a chair are certainly not good for overall muscle tone. Always consult with your physician, however, before enrolling in *any* exercise program.

If the goal of a rehabilitation program is to improve general fitness, to help the patient's frame of mind (to show the patient that he or she is *not* a cardiac cripple) and perhaps to prepare the patient for a return to a particularly demanding job, then one cannot argue with their objectives. What about the effect on preventing repeat heart attacks and death? There have been four large-scale trials to evaluate these end points. One took place in the United States (the National Exercise and Heart Disease Project), one in Canada (the Ontario Study) and two in Scandinavia (a Finnish study and the Gotenberg Trial in Sweden). Some of these studies suggest a benefit provided by rehabilitation programs in preventing recurrences and early death, but often the drop-out rate for these trials is too high to allow definite conclusions to be drawn. Even many of the patients who do not drop out do not adhere to the design protocol for one reason or another. Some of the reasons for poor adherence can be due to a change in the patient's medical conditions: symptoms become worse, and surgery is needed, etc. Other times, new symptoms or a change in existing symptoms prevent continuation of a training program. Sometimes the reason is lack of support from the spouse or family. And finally, there is always the problem of confounding factors when benefits are evaluated. Do those patients who seem to benefit from a training program do so because of the training *per se*, or because they stopped smoking or took medications for their high blood pressure, etc.? At this point, the cardiologist simply doesn't know.

The reader may now ask: Assuming that exercise and training are helpful, why is this so? What are the mechanisms by which physical activity benefits the heart? Aerobic exercise (exercise in which the muscles use oxygen) is the preferred type of exercise. When the muscle cell runs out of oxygen, it turns to other energy sources such as fatty acids; this is called non-aerobic exercise. Most aerobic exercises are dynamic; isotonic is the more physiologic term. The important concept to remember with dynamic exercise is that large muscles or muscle groups (the leg muscles, for example) are rhythmically contracting and relaxing with constant intensity (as in walking, swimming, biking). As the exercised muscles use oxygen at a steady rate, the respiratory and circulatory systems can replenish the supply and keep the cycle going. Obviously, if kept up long enough, even at a moderate rate, the oxygen supply will be depleted but, on the whole, most of the dynamic exercise is aerobic in nature. On the other hand, rapid, concentrated bursts of energy use up oxygen more quickly. If the exercise is dynamic, this may not necessarily be harmful (for example, running sprints instead of a slower jog). Dynamic exercise causes blood vessels to dilate rather than contract, thus increasing blood flow and reducing blood pressure. Because of this, some hypertensive patients can be treated with exercise programs alone. If an exercise is static, it can be harmful. Static exercises are the opposite of dynamic. They are also called isometric—the opposite of isotonic. There is not much body movement, but there is a lot of muscle contraction as parts of the body strain against a fixed resistance. A perfect example is weight lifting. Much of the muscular contraction in snow shoveling is isometric—this contributes to snow shoveling heart attacks. Not only are you rapidly using oxygen, but you are increasing your blood pressure—the exact opposite of what occurs in dynamic exercise.

Dr. Peter D. Wood reported in 1986, summarizing a 1984 NIH Workshop on Physical Activity and Fitness, that people who engage in endurance sports have lower concentrations of low-density lipoprotein cholesterol (the "bad" cholesterol) and higher concentrations of the "good" high-density lipoprotein cholesterol. This is not true for persons who engage in mostly non-aerobic training activities such as weight lifting. The beneficial effect of dynamic exercise can be seen with as little as 10 miles of running per week, or its equivalent. Three good 30 minute workouts per week can do the trick.

Because people who exercise regularly are more aware of their bodies, they tend to watch their diets more and smoke less —all to the good of the heart! Exercise may also lead to an improvement in the body's abilities to dissolve blood clots, but this has not been proven. There is evidence that in animal models (monkeys and rats) less severe degrees of coronary artery disease develop in those animals who are regularly exercised despite being fed special high-fat diets. For example, in 1981, Dr. D. M. Kramsch and colleagues from the Boston University Medical Center reported their studies on three groups of young monkeys. One group ate a normal diet, the second group ate a high-fat diet designed to produce coronary artery disease and the third group started on the normal diet then switched to the high-fat diet. The monkeys in the third group also ran on a treadmill for one hour three times per week throughout the three year trial. Some of the monkeys in the second group developed electrocardiographic changes, coronary artery disease and sudden death; but not the exercising monkeys nor the control monkeys in Group 1. Autopsy reports in the monkeys on high-fat diets showed that the exercising monkeys (Group 3) had larger caliber coronary arteries, with fewer fatty deposits, than did the non-exercising monkeys on the high-fat diet (Group 2). Obviously, what happens in a monkey may not happen in a human being, but these results support the concept that exercise benefits the heart.

RISKS OF EXERCISE

Some forms of exercise pose specific problems because of wear and tear on ligaments, joints, etc. Unfortunately, running is one of these types of exercise. We still don't know what the long term effects of moderate distance running will be in terms of future orthopedic problems. Bicycling, swimming and walking are less of a problem in this regard.

There are also risks to the heart involved in running, especially to people with known heart disease, but there are enough reports of apparently healthy runners dropping dead (the Jim Fixx syndrome in one variation or another) to also merit concern for this group. It is probable that many of these apparently healthy individuals had pre-existing but silent heart disease and that the exertion associated with their physical activity did them in. Data have been presented in previous chapters correlating electrocardiographic changes on exercise testing to underlying coronary artery disease. *All persons above the age of 35— especially men— who are about to engage in moderate to strenuous physical fitness programs and who have either a family history of heart disease or risk factors should first consult their physician about having an exercise electrocardiogram.* We realize that even in this high-risk group not all coronary artery disease will be detected by an exercise test and, conversely, that there will be some false-positive electrocardiograms, but there are ways to maximize the test results to achieve a good degree of reliablity. These include evaluation of risk factors in addition to the degree of ST depression. A screening electrocardiogram is *not* a panacea—some individuals will pass the test and then die running, others will fail the test and require radioisotopic tests to show that they are free of disease—but for most of us, it can be an enormous help.

When exercise does cause problems, one of those problems is cardiac arrhythmias (irregularities of the heartbeat). For example, during dynamic exercise in patients with known heart disease, the incidence of dangerous arrhythmias (such as ventricular tachycardia) can range from 2–5%; during static exercise, it can be as much as 15%. On the other hand, in apparently healthy and well-trained runners, ventricular tachycardia is very rare. Sudden death (presumably an arrhythmic event) during dynamic exercise can occur, but sudden death during static exercise—or a combination of static and dynamic exercise—is more common. Thus, in the week following a blizzard in Massachusetts, the death rate for coronary artery disease jumped markedly due to the amount of snow shoveling.

Some of the studies seem to show that sudden death is more likely to occur at higher rather than lower levels of exertion. Strenuous exercise may protect against development of heart disease, but when cardiac arrest occurs, it is more likely to occur during strenuous exercise! If one analyzes the data more carefully, this is not really so much of a paradox. Autopsy data on runners who die suddenly during exertion—and this includes marathon runners—show advanced degrees of coronary artery disease. (They probably had it before they even started running). Thus, in someone who already has disease, the protective effect of exercise may be minimal or nil. In some cases, it may be decidedly negative. In other words, as Dr. Edward Eichner stated so well in a 1983 report, "Exercise probably protects against heart disease, but sudden exertion can kill persons with heart disease."

To exercise or not to exercise? What is the consensus of the experts? We spoke again to Dr. William Kannel of the Boston University Medical Center, who was for many years medical director of the Framingham Study. "True, there is no reliably hard evidence that exercise protects against heart disease, and I'm not sure that physical inactivity is a separate risk factor. However, the evidence from around the world seems to suggest that regular physical activity appears to decrease the risk of coronary artery disease. It helps to control the conventional risk factors by making the participants pay more attention to their health (they have a more positive 'body image'), as well as by favorable physiologic effects (controlling blood pressure, weight, and so on)."

We would agree with this formulation. Modest exercise that can be readily performed by most people will probably not result in major orthopedic problems and may help prevent the development of coronary artery disease. It is not a vaccine; it does not confer immunity. Once disease is present, there is very little evidence that exercise will cause plaques within the blood vessels to get smaller, and, indeed, for some people exercise may be harmful. A word of warning: Consult with your physician first. An exercise test prior to an exercise program may be indicated, as we have mentioned earlier.

Having said all that, what do we recommend as a sensible, moderate exercise program? Although it is not clear that you need to become cardiovascularly conditioned or "trained" (in the physiological definition of the term) to achieve the presumed benefits of physical exercise, why not attempt to achieve this conditioning? The cost in time and effort to the person involved is not that much, and this is where the beneficial effect on controlling the conventional risk factors may be most striking. After an exercise program of a month's duration, your resting heart rate (taken after sitting quietly for several minutes) should no longer be the 72 beats per minute or so it was a month earlier—it should be in the 60s. To take your pulse, you needn't count for a whole minute: 15 or 30 seconds will do, then multiply by 4 or 2. Those who train vigorously will achieve even lower rates.

Our pulse rates are in the 50s; we average 20–30 miles a week of jogging at a rate of 8.5–10 miles per hour. Don't be discouraged if your heart rate only shows minimal changes at first—each person responds at his or her own pace. It may take months to decline fully. The important thing is not to give up the training program because changes aren't occurring fast enough.

At this point in the book, we would like to make some recommendations concerning a heart-healthy exercise program. These represent merely useful guidelines; they are not meant to be comprehensive. (For the reader interested in more detailed descriptions of fitness programs and caloric expenditures per activity, there are any number of commercially available books that can supply this information.) There are four major types of dynamic exercise that we recommend. The best from the orthopedic point of view is swimming because it causes no wear and tear on joints and ligaments. But it does require access to a pool year round. Cycling is good exercise but, for many individuals in urban settings, this poses logistic problems. These problems can be solved with an indoor, stationary bicycle positioned in front of a television set or a stereo amplifier (to fight the boredom factor). Jogging has been an "in thing" for several years, and we think it will remain that way because even urban dwellers have some access to parks or indoor running tracks. While professional tracks are best on the legs, asphalt surfaces are fine. Concrete is too hard on the legs, and grass may hide potentially dangerous crevices, stones, etc. Walking is an excellent substitute: walk to work, if possible; take stairs and not elevators; go for walks in the morning or evening. Explore new cities when you visit them—or the city you live in! The problem with walking is that most of us don't regard it as an exercise and do not do it regularly enough. Although for some persons it may lack the psychological benefits of a regular exercise program, we urge the public to walk whenever possible. For many individuals it can serve very well as *the* prime conditioning vehicle. Wear comfortable shoes with soft soles whenever possible. Sports? Sure, sports are fine, but as we will demonstrate, physical fitness depends on regular activity. Sports may not be that regular. Think of sports as leisure time activities to be enjoyed for their own sake. Of course, if you can play tennis for an hour a day, four days a week, there is also a fitness factor involved. The trick is to expend at least 300 calories per session, as we will describe subsequently.

Let's use jogging as an example. The three elements to the cardiovascular conditioning program are sometimes called the exercise prescriptions. They are *intensity*, *duration*, and *frequency*. Duration and frequency are easier to explain. Start with periods that last about 15 minutes and work up to 30 minutes or more. Unless you're in training for a specific event, like a marathon, there's little to be gained by more than an hour of jogging. Frequency is also simple: three or four sessions per week will suffice. This will insure a weekly caloric expenditure in excess of what is needed. Intensity is more difficult to explain. The goal is to eventually exercise at a heart rate that is about 75% of the maximal expected for someone your age. At the beginning, slightly less is acceptable. As a rough guide, the following heart rates are suggested as minimum: age 30, 136 beats per minute (estimated by taking your own pulse); age 35, 132; age 40, 128; age 45, 124; age 50, 119; age 55, 115; age 60, 111; age 65, 107. Once you achieve the target heart rate, try to continue to maintain it at that level. At the beginning, a 1-mile walk may suffice; after several weeks, a 3-mile run may be needed. Since heart rates are not that easy to calculate while exercising, a rule of thumb is that a rate sufficient to produce good cardiovascular stress will also produce a goodly amount of perspiration! If you haven't broken into a sweat, you're either not going a great enough distance, or you're doing it too slowly. After a month of running, 8.5–12 minute-miles should present no problems. Stopping exercise for three weeks for any reason undoes all your efforts, but one can start again. Cutting back to once a week has the same negative effect. In the final analysis, a cardiovascular conditioning program is either maintained or it isn't.

Another rule of thumb is used for the caloric expenditure involved in running. Running 1 mile in 10 minutes uses up about 100 calories. Briskly walking the same distance almost equals that caloric expenditure, even though it may take twice as long. (Carrying 2- or 3-pound weights in each hand while gently swinging your arms will increase the amount of calories burned.) The advantage of running over walking is in time saved, but if your job—or leisure time activities—involves considerable walking and this enables you to achieve a cardiovascular conditioning effect, so be it. Biking is another recommended activity, but if you bike at moderate speed, it will take you about 2.5 miles to burn up 100 calories.

All this exercise: Will it make you feel better, psychologically and physically? Yes. Will it help you lose weight? A little, but not much; that comes at the dining table. Will it open up new blood vessels (collaterals) in your heart? Probably not, despite what some wishful thinkers have postulated. The only stimulus for collateral growth is not enough flow to the heart in the first place! So if your vessels aren't blocked, collaterals don't form.

Should you be concerned if your heart walls become thicker, a so-called athlete's heart? First of all, this is not harmful as was once thought. Second, it is unlikely that recreational exercise will bring it about. In any event, the slower the heart rate at rest, the less blood your heart needs, regardless of its thickness. The most important effect of exercise, however, is not on the heart *per se* but on the circulation of the whole body (the systemic circulation). A lowered blood pressure and heart rate make fewer demands on the heart; the widened caliber of the coronary arteries should also make obstruction by plaques less likely. Should you only exercise in the afternoon or evening rather than the morning? We bring this point up because of data showing that heart attacks are more frequent in the morning (see Chapter 11). If you have no cardiac symptoms or risk factors (or have had a normal exercise test) you can exercise whenever you choose, but if you've had a heart attack there is more reason for concern. However, a study published in the *Archives of Internal Medicine* in 1993 found a low incidence of cardiac events in such patients no matter when they exercised. But, please, take your medicines first!

Whenever you exercise, remember, for the least trauma to your body muscles start off your dynamic exercise slowly, allow yourself five minutes to *warm up* by exercising at a slower pace and similarly about five minutes to *cool down* by doing the same thing. Stay away from static exercises . . . unless, of course, you're training to be a professional body builder. Weight lifting has its dangers, so see your doctor first!

10

Medical and Surgical Treatment of Heart Disease

The first line of treatment for most people with heart disease includes three types of drugs in addition to aspirin: nitrates, beta blockers, and calcium blockers. (The beta blockers and calcium blockers are also useful in treating high blood pressure.) The newest non-surgical technique for treating heart disease is called balloon angioplasty and involves mechanical widening of the narrowed coronary artery with a special catheter. Laser angioplasty and directional coronary atherectomy are even newer refinements of this technique. When non-surgical therapy fails, or when the disease is too extensive and/or life-threatening, coronary artery surgery has proven to be a generally safe and effective procedure.

Lancet, the leading medical journal in Great Britain, published a letter to the editor in its March 12, 1977 issue which led to a profound alteration in the way patients with coronary artery disease are treated. This remarkable letter—a rather unique way of presenting a medical breakthrough, to say the least—was the report of the first five successful procedures of balloon dilatation (stretching open) of blockages in human coronary arteries. The author of the letter was Dr. Andreas Gruntzig, a young Swiss cardiologist. For several years, Dr. Gruntzig had been intrigued with investigative reports about the use of special catheters that could be used to open narrowings in leg arteries. After careful experiments in animals dilating blockages in legs, kidneys, and coronary arteries, and after experiences in humans with athero-sclerotic blockages in legs and other arteries, Dr. Gruntzig was ready to try the technique on human coronary arteries for the first time. His success in the small, initial series of patients was followed by successful dilatations in thousands of others! No discussion of heart disease therapy today is complete without inclusion of percutaneous transluminal coronary angioplasty (PTCA), as the procedure is technically called. And it was first published as a letter to the editor!

In this chapter, we will update developments in treating heart disease: first with drugs, then with PTCA and its "first cousins" laser angioplasty and directional coronary atherectomy, and, lastly, with surgery. *The very important issue of whether women are denied appropriate access to these drugs and proce- dures (either before or after heart attacks) is discussed separately in Chapter 13.*

DRUG THERAPY

There are three classes of drugs that are particularly useful in coronary heart disease. They are, in order of appearance on the medical scene, the nitrates, the beta-blocking drugs, and the calcium-blocking drugs. We will also have a few words to say about new indications for the use of that ubiquitous drug, aspirin.

Nitrates were described by the English physician T.L. Brun- ton over 100 years ago in 1867. The most widely used prepa- ration is the "under-the-tongue" pill, nitroglycerin. Taken in this manner, the drug is rapidly absorbed into the bloodstream through the large veins on the bottom surface of the tongue. Cardiac effects occur in two to three minutes. Other nitrate preparations are made to be swallowed and prevent attacks from occurring. These include isosorbide dinitrate (brand names Isordil and Sorbitrate). Nitroglycerin ointment, which is placed on the skin (brand names Deponit, Minitran, Nitro-Dur, Transderm-Nitro, Nitro-Bid, Nitrol, and Nitrodisc), is also available. Isosorbide dinitrate pills are taken three times a day, the ointment several times a day or once a day as a "patch." Side effects are flushing and dizziness, with headaches reported by some patients. The newest oral preparation is isosorbide mononitrate, a more active form of the drug (brand name Ismo, which is taken twice daily). One word of caution about oral and transdermal nitrates: if taken *too* often, tolerance develops and the drug loses its potency, so follow the prescribed guidelines carefully. One of the attractive features about isosorbide mononitrate is its ready availability in the blood stream. When used as directed, tolerance is abolished while the drug's cardiac effects remain.

How do these drugs work? They relax the muscular layer in the walls of blood vessels, thereby dilating (expanding) the channel through which blood passes. It is now known that once in the body the nitrates are broken down to nitric oxide, a powerful dilator substance that is the chemical equivalent of the body's own vasodilator, termed endothelium derived relaxing factor or EDRF. When the interior lining of the blood vessels are injured (as they are in atherosclerosis), EDRF production decreases, resulting in additional narrowing of the vessel. The nitrates can blunt this effect.

Dilating the narrowings in the coronary arteries and their branches means a better blood supply to the heart and less ischemia. Just as importantly, the nitrates also dilate veins and arteries throughout the body. With a person in the upright position, this effect causes pooling of blood in the feet and legs, slowing the return of blood to the heart and reducing its workload. Less work means less need for oxygen; the harmful effects of blockages in the coronary arteries are minimized.

When should these drugs be taken? As we indicated, nitroglycerin is the drug of choice to treat chest pain, but many patients are not aware that the under-the-tongue preparation is also very useful in *preventing* an anginal episode just before it would otherwise occur. For example, if taken 10-15 minutes before an activity known to cause angina in a particular patient (sexual activity, for example), angina will *not* occur most of the time. Another important bit of advice is to take nitroglycerin while sitting up rather than standing or lying flat. Standing is not advised because dilation of arteries all over the body may cause a fall in blood pressure leading to dizziness or even a fainting spell. Lying flat also creates problems because when a person lies down, the legs are no longer in a dependent position thus preventing the "pooling" effect on the venous circulation. The message? If you need to take this medication, sit; don't lie down or stand up.

Nitrates were the first type of anti-anginal drugs used to treat silent ischemia. In the late 1970s, Dr. Carl Pepine of the University of Florida combined administration of nitrates with his early Holter monitor studies of patients with angina. "It made sense to us that a drug like nitroglycerin, which affects both 'supply and demand' would reduce ischemic events, and it did, dramatically." In these studies, hourly administration of nitroglycerin markedly decreased both angina and silent ischemia. Although it is not convenient for patients to take the drug in this manner, today Dr. Pepine feels the same effects can be achieved with a combination of nitrates and other drugs taken by mouth one or more times each day. This approach has been validated by research studies performed in many centers.

Beta blockers were introduced in Europe in the lates 1950s, but like so many new drugs did not receive United States Food and Drug Administration approval until much later. They are called beta blockers because of their physiologic actions on the beta receptors (biochemical binding sites) that are found in heart tissue, blood vessel walls, and in other parts of the body including the lungs and uterus. The beta receptors, with their "cousins" the alpha receptors, are so named because they are thought to moderate the specific alpha and beta properties of those hormones involved in "fight or flight" situations. These hormones are epinephrine and norepinephrine (also called adrenalin and noradrenalin). As we described in Chapter 5, these hormones are vital in preparing the body for sudden bouts of extreme exertion. The alpha receptors are responsible for blood vessels constricting and for small breathing tubes in the lungs dilating. The beta receptors do the opposite of the alpha receptors, so that the body's functions are always in balance—though the balance may shift one way or the other in acute situations.

The beta receptors found in special areas of heart tissue are responsible for the heart rate speeding up under certain circumstances. By lowering the heart rate, the beta blockers can relieve or prevent ischemia. As we noted earlier, reducing a person's heart rate from 72 to 50 beats per minute, for example—will sharply reduce the amount of oxygen needed by the heart muscle to function effectively. Therefore, if there is a partial blockage in a blood vessel and that blockage restricts the blood flow to the heart, the beta-blocking drug will not eliminate the blockage, but it can minimize its destructiveness by reducing the heart's need for oxygen. Thus, the reduced amount of oxygen carried in the blood passing through the blockage will now be sufficient to meet the heart's oxygen demand. Beta blockers are particularly helpful when ischemic episodes are related to exertion: the higher the heart rate at which chest pain ensues, the more effective the beta blocker will be. Preventing the heart rate from reaching that critical point—the ischemic threshold—can also reduce the frequency and severity of painful episodes.

Eight of these drugs are now approved by the Food and Drug Administration. Propranolol (brand name Inderal) is the oldest. Others include metoprolol (Lopressor), atenolol (Tenormin), pindolol (Visken), nadolol (Corgard), acebutolol (Sectral) and labetalol (Trandate, Normodyne). Many studies have been done in patients to validate the anti-ischemic effects of these drugs. In summary, it can be said that in general, these drugs are well tolerated and do exactly what they are supposed to do—reduce the number of anginal attacks and improve the ability to exercise without having chest pain. We and others have also seen them markedly reduce the frequency of silent ischemia.

The variety of beta-blocking drugs enables the physician to tailor the medication to the needs of the patient. Is a once-a-day preparation called for? Atenolol and nadolol only have to be given once a day, and there is now also a sustained long-acting release preparation of propranolol and metoprolol. These long-acting drugs are often satisfactory for many angina sufferers, and they are ideally suited for those who also need treatment of high blood pressure.

In addition to treating angina, several of the drugs (propranolol, atenolol, timolol, and metoprolol) have been shown to have a protective effect *after* a heart attack. The very large Beta Blocker Heart Attack Trial or BHAT study in the United States and European trials involving atenolol, metoprolol and timolol were landmark studies in this area (see Chapter 11). In the Beta Blocker Heart Attack Trial, propranolol was administered 7–21 days after the heart attack and reduced the one year mortality rate by 25% compared to the rate for patients receiving a placebo. Side effects of these drugs include fatigue, mental depression, gastrointestinal upset, and constriction of the breathing tubes. Because of the last effect, they are *never* to be used in asthmatics. They are also not to be used in patients with slow heart rates or severe heart failure associated with fluid build-up in the feet and lungs, since they can make both of these conditions worse. Sudden withdrawal of these drugs, for unclear reasons, can also cause a rebound increase in chest pain.

Like the nitrates, the *calcium blockers* dilate blood vessels by relaxing the muscular layers in the walls of the blood vessels. However, their method of action is related to their effect on the movement of calcium from one part of the muscle cell in the wall of the vessel to another part of the cell. This movement of calcium triggers the muscle cell contraction. Other terms used to describe calcium blockers are calcium channel blockers and calcium antagonists.

At the present time, there are five calcium blockers approved by the Food and Drug Administration. They are nifedipine (trade names Procardia and Adalat) and two brand new derivatives, amlodipine (Norvasc) and felodipine (Plendil), as well as verapamil (Calan and Isoptin) and diltiazem (Cardizem and Dilacor). In clinical trials from around the world, these drugs have been convincingly shown to reduce the frequency and intensity of angina attacks in patients with atherosclerotic blockages in their coronary arteries. Most attention has, of course, been paid to those episodes associated with chest pain. This is not surprising in light of our earlier discussions indicating that the acceptance of silent heart disease as a real entity is a comparatively recent event. However, there is also data that calcium blockers help silent ischemia as well.

In one of the most important clinical studies with these drugs, Dr. Elliott Antman and colleagues from the Harvard Medical School were able to show the effectiveness of the most commonly used type, nifedipine, in patients with a syndrome known as Prinzmetal's angina. This syndrome is characterized by the coronary arteries becoming completely obstructed by spasm; that is, intense contraction in the muscular walls of the artery causes complete obstruction of the central opening of the vessel (the lumen). These patients have an especially difficult time since the occurrence of the spasm attack is often completely unpredictable. Interestingly, they almost always occur when patients are *not* exerting themselves. (By contrast, most patients with angina have ischemia with exertion; others have it both when at rest and with exertion). In Dr. Antman's study, reported in 1980, 127 patients were studied in several different hospitals, all of which followed a standard protocol. All patients had previous treatment with conventional anti-anginal therapy with disappointing results. In a remarkable turnabout, addition of nifedipine caused total elimination of the painful attacks in 63% of the patients. In another 24%, the number of attacks decreased by at least half.

Side effects severe enough to require withdrawal of the drug occurred in only 5% of the patients. These side effects included headache, flushing, and dizziness—all related to the drug's effect of dilating blood vessels. Such effects are similar to those seen with the nitrates. Unique to calcium blockers, however, is the occasional development of leg edema (fluid build-up), a local effect not related to heart failure. This usually clears after treatment with diuretics (water pills).

The impressive results that nifedipine achieved in the patients with Prinzmetal's angina—as well as in those with other forms of angina—suggested that it would be effective in any situation where increased blood vessel constriction might be a factor. With this background, it is not surprising that the drug has also been used successfully in patients with frequent episodes of both angina and silent ischemia. The goal is to reduce all ischemic episodes (the "total ischemic burden").

Diltiazem and verapamil are not as potent vasodilators as nifedipine, but they both possess one feature that nifedipine does not: they slow the heart rate by a mechanism similar to that of the beta blockers. It must be re-emphasized that this effect of slowing the heart is very important for patients with angina. The reason for this is that the slower the heart rate, the less oxygen the heart needs for its pumping activity, and therefore the less likely it is that ischemia will ensue. In clinical trials, these drugs have been shown to reduce the number of angina episodes per day and to improve exercise tolerance in a manner similar to that described for nifedipine. Like nifedipine, these drugs can be given three or four times per day, but all are now available in long-acting preparations to be given once or twice a day.

Studies using verapamil in patients with angina and silent myocardial ischemia were reported in 1986. Dr. Oberdan Paroldi and his colleagues in Pisa, Italy, were able to reduce both the number of painful and silent episodes with this particular calcium blocker. Verapamil's side effects are related to its slowing of the heart rate and it is more powerful than diltiazem in this regard. Many physicians do not use it in patients who already have slow intrinsic heart rates, or in patients who are already receiving beta blockers, because these drugs also slow the heart rate.

Contrary to popular belief, there are not a lot of drugs (besides the ones mentioned) that are helpful in treating myocardial ischemia. Drugs that control the heart's rhythm (anti-arrhythmics, like quinidine) are only useful when there is an abnormality in the rhythm. Similarly, drugs that cause the heart to beat more forcefuly—like digitalis—are only helpful when the heartbeat is sluggish, and excess water has built up in the feet and lungs.

In one of the ironic twists that sometimes occur in the medical world, aspirin, the old standby of the family medicine chests, has been shown to reduce the frequency of subsequent heart attacks in some people who have angina or have had a prior heart attack. The most recent study published in 1992 by a Swedish group shows that aspirin can also reduce mortality in silent ischemia patients. How does aspirin work? In low doses (for example, one adult table per day, or 325mg) it blocks the tendency for small blood particles, platelets, to clump together in the lumens of diseased blood vessels and obliterate the blood channel. By contrast, conventional blood thinners (anticoagulants) have not been shown to be useful in reducing heart attacks. Whether the drugs work especially well in larger doses is unclear, but the incidence of gastrointestinal complications, especially stomach bleeding, increases markedly as the dosage increases. To be on the safe side, take no more than 325mg of aspirin per day. For headaches, arthritis, etc., take other medications.

PERCUTANEOUS TRANSLUMINAL CORONARY ANGIOPLASTY (PTCA) AND RELATED PROCEDURES

PTCA is now a standard non-surgical technique for the treatment of angina (and in some cases, heart attacks). As we noted at the beginning of this chapter, this procedure was devised by the late Dr. Andreas Gruntzig in 1977, who was unfortunately killed in a plane crash several years later. The angioplasty procedure uses a special catheter with a distensible balloon near its tip. Inserted in a partially blocked blood vessel, the balloon is inflated and presses the atherosclerotic plaque against the vessel wall. (Fig. D). This makes the channel wider and allows the increase of the previously restricted blood flow. Trials of patients with angina who have been treated with PTCA show that this is

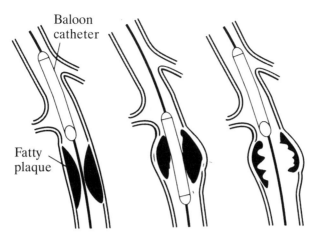

Figure D
The balloon angioplasty procedure: A balloon catheter is inserted into an artery narrowed by fatty deposits; the balloon is inflated to push the fatty tissue outward; the balloon is deflated and removed, leaving a larger opening through which blood can more easily pass.

often an effective way of managing their illness. In many instances, the opened blood vessel remains that way for years, but in about a third it will close again, usually within a year. Serious complications from the procedure itself occur in less than 5% of patients and can require emergency coronary artery bypass surgery.

The number of these procedures is skyrocketing. In 1991, over 300,000 balloon angioplasties were performed in the United States alone, compared to 400,000 coronary bypass operations! Initial success rates approach 90% in many of the more experienced centers, even though they are treating more patients with complicated anatomy. Who undergoes PTCA? Usually patients who would otherwise undergo surgery. However, not all surgical candidates can have PTCA. The blockages must be accessible to the PTCA catheter.

Newer techniques have been combined with conventional balloon angioplasty. One such technique uses laser beams to vaporize plaques. Another technique employs devices at the tip of the angioplasty catheter to shell out parts of the blockage (rotational atherectomy and directional coronary atherectomy). Are these advances truly an improvement over conventional PTCA? In some patients the answer is clearly yes, and this is where they are used most extensively. Unfortunately, the re-occlusion rate is still about one in three, even for the new procedures.

Recently, PTCA has been adapted for use in patients in the early hours of a heart attack—a truly exciting breakthrough. This is discussed further in Chapter 11.

ENHANCED EXTERNAL COUNTERPULSATION (EECP)

In the late 1960s, a heart surgeon in Boston invented a device to help get an additional blood supply to diseased heart muscle during heart attacks. This circulation assist device of William Birtwell and Dr. Harry Soroff resembled the bottom half of an astronaut's suit connected to an air pump. The inflation-deflation sequence of the gravity-suit boosted the return of blood to the heart during the resting part of the heart's cycle (diastole). In the 1970s and 1980s, Dr. Zhen Zheng at Sun Yat Sen School of Medicine—realizing that China had limited re-sources for high technology medical procedures such as PTCA and cardiac surgery—improved the design of the Birtwell-Soroff device and used it on thousands of patients with angina. Thanks to Dr. Soroff's efforts, the device made its way to our experi-mental research laboratory at Stony Brook in the late 1980s. In a study published in 1992, it was shown to be effective in treating "end-stage" angina patients, i.e., those who had failed drugs, PTCA and/or coronary surgery. In nearly all patients the treat-ment strikingly reduced or eliminated the angina. As a result, the Sun Yat Sen School of Medicine and a public company (Future Medical Products, Inc. of New York) established a joint venture to make this device available to angina patients in the United States. In Britain, where long waits for elective cardiac surgery are common, a unique series of studies are planned to see if EECP can be used as a "first-line" treatment to either avoid or delay the need for cardiac surgery. The medical and economic implications of the effectiveness of such a noninvasive approach are enormous, and we will be watching the British tests with great interest.

CORONARY ARTERY BYPASS SURGERY

There have been many different operations attempted for patients with angina over the past 30 years. Some of these operations involved cutting the nerves to the heart. Pain was often relieved, but obviously the natural history of the disease was not affected. The arteries supplying the heart muscle were still blocked, and the heart still did not receive enough blood flow when under a severe enough workload. Other operations were designed to improve blood flow to the heart. The idea of improving the blood supply was the right one, but initial operations aimed at doing so did not deliver enough blood to improve the situation. Some of these procedures sound very odd today! For example, opening the chest and applying an irritant like sterile talcum powder to the external surface of the heart caused the surface to adhere to the lining around the heart (the pericardium) and stimulated new vessel growth between the pericardium and the heart. Unfortunately for the makers of talcum powder, not only was the new vessel growth inadequate, but it occurred in the outermost layers of the heart muscle rather than in the deeper layers where it was needed the most.

In 1964, the Canadian surgeon Dr. Arthur Vineberg reported on a new and more physiologic approach. He connected the artery from beneath the breast bone into the heart muscle itself. Because heart muscle has tiny spaces between fiber bundles, there is room for new vessels to grow from the "implanted" artery. This operation achieved moderate success and paved the way for other procedures that permitted an even greater increase in blood flow. The Cleveland Clinic was instrumental in introducing or popularizing many of the procedures, but Dr. Michael DeBakey's turned out to be the most effective one. Working in Houston, he took a vein from the leg of a patient, attached one end to a coronary artery and attached the other end to the aorta (Fig. E). Over time, this is the only surgical procedure that has proven completely successful from both a clinical and physiological perspective. Because the vein from the leg (or, alternatively, the internal mammary artery lying behind the breast bone) is connected from the main artery of the body (the aorta) to the coronary artery beyond the obstruction, blood flow "bypasses" the obstruction.

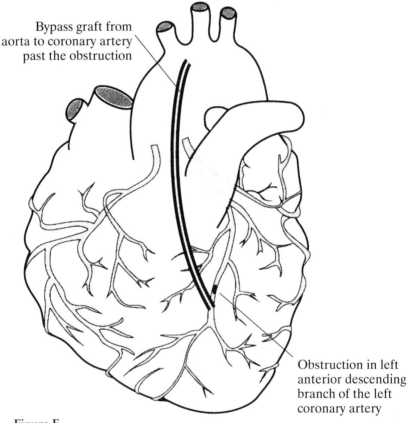

Bypass graft from aorta to coronary artery past the obstruction

Obstruction in left anterior descending branch of the left coronary artery

Figure E
The coronary bypass operation: Lying on the outer surface of the left ventricle are an obstructed coronary artery and a venous bypass graft from the aorta to the coronary artery beyond the obstruction.

Reasons for recommending surgery are primarily based on relief of pain, but in some instances the extent and severity of the blockages are reason enough to operate. For example, the large, multicentered studies (discussed in Chapter 5) from the United States and Europe found that blockage of the main left coronary artery should be treated surgically. These studies compared survival in operated and non-operated patients in order to reach that conclusion. In the opinion of many cardiologists, other types of extensive disease (so-called triple-vessel disease) are also grounds for operation even in minimally symptomatic patients. This is even true for some asymptomatic patients, especially if they have had a heart attack in the past. In 1985, the multicenter Coronary Artery Surgery Study (CASS) found that patients who were asymptomatic after their heart attacks but who had severe disease involving all three major coronary arteries and some impairment of the heart's pumping ability had only about a 1% per year mortality if operated upon—compared to 5% per year mortality in the non-operated patients. As noted, patients with obstruction of the main left coronary artery are also usually recommended for surgery, regardless of the degree of symptoms. Ample documentation shows the potential damage from such a blockage is a "widow-maker."

Even when the coronary bypass operation is successful, the long-term results are still in doubt. About 20% of the vein grafts, and a smaller percentage of the breast bone arteries, will close by the end of the first year following surgery. Each year a small number of the remaining grafts also close totally or partially. As a result about 3% of patients per year experience recurrence of symptoms over a 5–10 year follow-up period. Other long-term problems include development of new obstructions either in non-operated vessels or beyond the area of surgery in operated vessels. Direct complications of surgery (death, heart attack) range from 1–5% depending on how sick the patient and how poorly the heart contracts. New York State has been a pioneer in maintaining a risk-adjusted mortality registry of the state's 30 cardiac surgical facilities. Data on individual surgeons is also available. Surgical risk should be discussed in detail with the patient's physician (and surgeon) before surgery is performed, but it must be emphasized that most of the 400,000 patients who have coronary bypass surgery each year experience no serious complications.

Having updated current treatment, what conclusions can we draw? Disease caused by fatty deposits in the coronary arteries is relentless; PTCA and surgery are palliative but not curative. Only measures to prevent the disease will be of long-term value. As we have seen in earlier chapters, these measures are best instituted before disease is present. Even when disease is already present, however, it is still essential to lower blood cholesterol, correct high blood pressure, and stop smoking. In many patients treatment with drugs, PTCA, or cardiac surgery will improve the quality of life and often prolong it. If EECP proves as beneficial as our early studies suggest, it could become an important adjunct to these other therapies.

How much has medical and surgical therapy been responsible for the decline in heart disease mortality in the United States? The best estimates of those who have analyzed this problem—including Dr. William Kannel of the Framingham Study and Dr. Lee Goldman and associates at the Brigham and Women's Hospital in Boston—are that changes in diet and lifestyle probably account for most of the decline, though a significant portion of the reduction can be ascribed to therapy.

CHAPTER

11

The Revolution in Heart Attack Treatment

The ability to open blocked coronary arteries during the early hours of a heart attack has dramatically changed the way many doctors treat heart attack victims. Special drugs are now available that can quickly dissolve blood clots, provided the patient comes to the hospital within 6-12 hours after the onset of chest pain. Alternatively, balloon angioplasty can be used to open the blockage and then "flatten" the residual fatty deposits in the blood vessels, thereby (hopefully) preventing future attacks. After the occurence of a heart attack, a variety of drugs are used to improve outcome, including beta blockers, aspirin, and a new class of drugs, the ACE-inhibitors.

A revolution has occurred in the treatment of heart attacks, but unfortunately, not enough physicians and patients are really aware of its implications. Traditionally, the heart attack victim was given morphine to stop his pain, while his physician reassured him that he would recover. Meanwhile, the physician checked for signs of treatable complications such as fluid buildup and irregular heartbeats. Other than that, the heart attack was left to run its course. For many patients, a "good" physician was the comforting grandfatherly type, much like the image of the family doctor sitting through the night holding a little girl's feverish hand in his own, while grateful parents looked on. More times than not, the child died. When the child recovered, it was probably due as much to her own resiliency as to the limited drugs available to the doctor. In 1993, this approach is outdated. You don't want only a warm, comforting type sitting by your bed if you have a heart attack; you want an aggressive, confident, well-trained cardiologist doing what needs to be done to eliminate the blockage in your coronary artery! A touch of gray at the temples can't hurt, nor can a little personality, but, in the final analysis, none of that matters if the doctor can save your heart!*

Why is it so important to be able to treat a heart attack aggressively? The answer is simple. Heart muscle (unlike some other parts of the body, like the skin) will not regenerate. Once a portion of the heart is gone, it is gone forever. The less heart muscle you have, the less effectively your heart beats and the less likely you are to have a normal life span—provided that you survive the heart attack in the first place. It is no longer good medical procedure to simply load patients with morphine until their blood-deprived heart muscle dies, and the pain finally stops. If the patient arrives early enough at the hospital, active intervention is possible.

There is probably nothing more catastrophic to the lay person than the thought of a heart attack. We quickly conjure up fears of death or long disability. But this need not be the case. Exciting new developments in the treatment of heart attacks have revolutionized the way doctors think of this problem.

The cause of a heart attack is straightforward enough—in most cases, a coronary artery becomes totally blocked, the blood supply to the affected area of heart muscle dries up, and the

---

*Occasionally the authors don't agree with each other. This is one such case. JKC disagrees with PFC and thinks that even in this setting, the personality of the doctor is very important!

muscle dies. When part of the heart dies, the end result can range from bad to awful. At a minimum, destruction of heart tissue is obviously not a plus for the patient. A two to three month period of convalescence is necessary before a return to full activity, and the patient will usually require some kind of conditioning program to strengthen the heart and keep body musculature in shape. There are also psychological problems associated with the interruption of one's normal activities and the fear of a recurrence.

If the heart attack is uncomplicated—that is, there is no residual pain, irregular heartbeat (arrhythmia), or buildup of fluid in the legs or other parts of the body—then the patient is relatively lucky. At the other extreme, the patient dies from the heart attack or is left with such weakened heart muscle that a return to useful activities is questionable and a normal life span may be severely threatened. It is imperative, therefore, to nip heart attacks in the bud whenever possible. How can this be accomplished?

Only about half the victims of a fatal or non-fatal heart attack will have prior warning—that is, transient symptoms of chest pain or pressure that warn patients that something is wrong and (we hope) send them to the doctor. Treating this angina will not necessarily guarantee the prevention of a heart attack, but at least it reduces the chances of an imminent attack. With definitive therapy—such as balloon angioplasty or coronary surgery—there is even a better chance preventing one in some patients with certain types of blockages.

For the other, less fortunate half of the heart attack victims, their first inkling that something is wrong will be the heart attack itself. A good portion of these people (perhaps as many as 60%) will never reach the hospital. As many as 400,000 people in the United States alone will die suddenly each year, most of them without reaching the hospital. Nearly all these deaths result from fatal heart arrhythmias. Mobile emergency teams can rescue some of the people if called quickly and if bystanders apply cardiopulmonary resuscitation immediately. After three minutes of oxygen deprivation, the human brain loses so much vital tissue that even if cardiac resuscitation is successful, the chances are great that the patient will wind up in a vegetative state.

Even though most angina comes on with exertion, most heart attacks are not related to exertion. In fact, there is no uniform pattern as to when heart attacks strike. Thanks largely to work reported by Dr. James Muller of Harvard Medical School, there is now a large body of evidence that heart attacks occur in a circadian variation, with peaks at 6 a.m. to noon and again at about 5 to 8 p.m. The explanation of the later peak is unclear, but the earlier and more important one seems clearly related to assuming the upright posture after long hours of reclining. There is a marked surge in certain hormones with resulting increases in narrowing of blood vessels and an increased propensity of the blood to clot. No matter when the episodes occur, however, symptoms may be vague. As we noted in Chapter 5, Dr. Muller feels strongly that there are certain "triggers" of heart attacks. Stressful activities, whether they be mental or physical, are such triggers. "Sometimes I think the public understands this concept better than do physicians," Dr. Muller told us.

The 40% of patients that do not die suddenly from their heart attack will often experience either chest pain, nausea, arm tingling, or other complaints as an indication of their heart attack. Those prudent enough to seek medical attention promptly can benefit greatly. Unfortunately for many individuals, this is a time when they procrastinate—denying that a heart attack could happen to them. Even physicians are guilty of this denial! We learn of too many cases of "indigestion" that turn out to be heart attacks in retrospect. In many instances, the discomfort of a heart attack—and angina, too, for that matter—resembles indigestion, is associated with belching, and is sometimes coincidentally relieved with antacids. It's better to err on the side of safety. A new sensation in the chest, arm, jaw, or even abdomen that suggests heart disease should receive medical attention.

Most of the public is not aware of this fact, which is another reason they pass off many complaints as indigestion. Chest discomfort (for that is what it usually is rather than pain per se) that persists for 20 minutes or more requires medical attention. Most people describe a heart attack as a severe ache that feels like a great weight on the chest; profuse sweating and difficulty in breathing are common accompaniments to the discomfort. If your own doctor is not available, go to the nearest hospital emergency room. If you don't think you can make it on your own, have someone take you. If the symptoms become worse, telephone for emergency assistance.

Once the emergency medical team arrives or the patient reaches a hospital emergency room, chances of survival increase enormously. Now the patient is in the hands of trained personnel who can treat dangerous heart irregularities quickly and efficiently. They will insert intravenous tubing while quickly performing an examination and hooking up an electrocardiogram. If the electrocardiogram shows telltale signs of an early heart attack, the patient will receive an intravenous injection of lidocaine (a powerful drug to treat irregular heartbeats) to prevent the occurence of a fatal heart rhythm disturbance (ventricular fibrillation). The installation of coronary care units (CCUs) in the 1960s resulted in a dramatic decline in hospital deaths from heart attacks due to ventricular fibrillation. Electrocardiographic monitors in every room, with satellite units at the nurses' stations, allow prompt electrocardiographic detection of dangerous ventricular arrhythmias that prevent adequate pumping of blood. As a result, reduction of deaths due to these arrhythmias have been the main accomplishment of these units. We can expect an even further reduction in these deaths now that magnesium infusions have been shown to dramatically reduce their incidence. This data comes from the results of several studies in Europe, as well as a "meta- analysis" published in the New England Journal of Medicine in 1992 that pooled the results of various studies. Although arrhythmic deaths have been reduced, deaths due to destruction of heart muscle have not been greatly affected by the CCUs. Even the advent of cardiac surgery did not appreciably reduce this total. The best treatment for *cardiogenic shock*, the medical name for the syndrome that results from massive destruction of the heart, is preventing such destruction from happening at all. But how can we do this once a heart attack has begun?

Until 1985, standard practice would be to admit heart attack patients, or suspected heart patients, to the CCU. In 1985, the United States Food and Drug Administration approved the use of a drug called streptokinase (brand names Streptase and Kabikinase) for dissolving clots in blood vessels. In the late 1970s research studies showed it was effective when injected directly into the blocked coronary artery, but this required performing coronary arteriography to pinpoint the clogged artery. Many centers with cardiac catheterization laboratories began using intracoronary streptokinase for the management of patients in the early stages of a heart attack. Their success rates in opening previously blocked coronary arteries prompted the Food and Drug Administration—not usually known for its speed in certifying new drugs—to approve intracoronary streptokinase for widespread (rather than only experimental) use. Therefore, instead of going to the CCU, a heart attack victim could go directly to the cardiac catheterization laboratory and have the blocked artery opened! The management of heart attacks thus underwent radical change. Where it was once considered dangerous to perform coronary arteriography in the early throes of a heart attack, it was now considered a therapeutic procedure. Fortunately, the most recent trials of *intravenous* streptokinase now show it to be nearly as effective as the intracoronary type. In 1987, the Food and Drug Administration approved its use. Intravenous treatment is preferred because it is easier and faster to administer and the key to the successful administration of streptokinase in *any* form is timing. Animal experiments indicated that if the blocked coronary artery could be re-opened within several hours of the occlusion it could minimize the damage from a heart attack. Many times it isn't possible to give intracoronary streptokinase and still be within the necessary time period (preferably no more than six hours and certainly no more than 12 from the onset of the pain). But all of these steps mean little if the patient arrives in the emergency room too late to receive this type of help—another key reason why denial of symptoms of a heart attack can be disastrous! Research estimates that only 25% of heart attack victims reach the hospital within the prescribed "window" of opportunity for clot busting and have no specific contraindications (such as recent stomach bleeding) for receiving the drugs.

The major problem with intravenous streptokinase is bleeding. The drug goes all over the body—not just to the heart—and because of its action on the blood clotting system in general, there is a threat of bleeding internally, as well as of bleeding under the skin. (This is akin to the situation facing a hemophiliac or patients taking blood-thinners for a variety of disease states.) In the final analysis, the risks of taking the drug are worthwhile because of the heart tissue it saves.

Given these risks of streptokinase, the next step was to find a compound that would break apart only fresh clots; in other words, a very specific agent that would minimize bleeding elsewhere in the body. Such a drug was prepared using new gene-splicing technology. It is called recombinant tissue plasminogen activator (rTPA or TPA or alteplase) and is marketed under the trade name Activase. When the Food and Drug Administration was made aware of the results of a large, multicentered Thrombolysis in Myocardial Infarction (TIMI) trial directed by Dr. Eugene Braunwald of the Harvard Medical School, it approved alteplase for use in 1988. This study has had many offshoots. Researchers assign patients randomly to treatment with rTPA, streptokinase, other clot-busters, or a placebo. They then further sub-divide each group, depending on whether patients undergo PTCA. These studies have already answered many questions about the correct approach to therapy of an early heart attack, and more is still to come.

Although intravenous clot-busters are successful in opening the blocked vessel in about 50–70% of cases, there is a significant re-occlusion rate within days or weeks. This is because there is a large atherosclerotic plaque sitting under the clot. Dissolving the clot does nothing to the plaque! Chances are that in many patients a clot will reform on the roughened edges of the plaque—it's just a question of time. Therefore, the next revolutionary step in the treatment of heart attacks was performing balloon angioplasty to flatten plaques, make vessel lumens wider, and reduce the possibility of re-occlusions. Angioplasty further emphasizes the need for hospitals with a cardiac catheterization laboratories. But what if the patient has no such facility nearby and is admitted to a local community hospital?

For the situation in which a cardiac catheterization laboratory is not available, intravenous clot-busters can be used and then the patient can be transferred elsewhere for the angioplasty procedure. This is not as difficult as it sounds.

There is a cardiac facility within hours of most community hospitals. A sensible approach is for community hospitals to "feed" their patients into the larger teaching centers. The experience of the cardiology group at the University of Michigan in Ann Arbor, deserves mention. In 1985 and 1986, under the directions of Drs. William O'Neill, Bertram Pitt and their colleagues, this group reported their experiences as a referral center for a large area in their state that is not geographically close to Ann Arbor. Whenever possible, the community hospital administers intravenous clot-busters to the patient. They are then brought by helicopter to Ann Arbor. If the vessel is opened and the residual plaque is small, no further therapy is instituted at the time. In one of Dr. O'Neill's recent reports, this only occurred in 3 of 34 patients. In 13 other patients, the streptokinase did not open the vessel. Emergency balloon angioplasty opened it in 12 of the 13. In 18 other patients, the vessel had opened but the residual plaque was large. Sixteen of these patients underwent balloon angioplasty, which successfully widened the vessel interiors.

What is the role of PTCA after a heart attack? Should it only be used if ischemia persists, as the TIMI trials suggest? The March 11, 1993, issue of the *New England Journal of Medicine* included three different articles on PTCA as a first-line treatment for acute heart attacks, accompanied by an editorial. The consensus was that immediate PTCA seems to be an attractive *alternative* to clot-busting drugs when the necessary facilities and personnel are available. This procedure should be considered for patients with contraindications to clot-busters (such as bleeding disorders), patients with massive heart attacks, and older people. The advantages of PTCA are that there is less chance of dangerous bleeding, and the patient is left with an "open artery," which in some studies at least predicts a better outcome in the long run.

Whether rTPA will replace intravenous streptokinase in the future remains to be seen, since it is more expensive than streptokinase ($2000 vs. $200). Seven large trials with strange sounding acronyms (ISIS, GISI, etc.) have not shown it to be superior, especially when combined with our old standby aspirin, but one trial (GUSTO) has. Some European trials even report success with either drug as much as 12–24 hours after the event. What about the patients with unrecognized or silent heart attacks? Obviously, this approach will not help, hence the need to identify potential victims before the attack and institute appropriate therapy that could prevent its occurrence.

After the heart attack, the patient's stay in the hospital is determined by several factors, including the occurence of a "non-Q-wave" rather than a "Q-wave" heart attack. A Q-wave infarction (an electrocardiographic term) occurs when the coronary artery supplying a section of heart muscle is totally blocked. Therefore, a non-Q-wave infarction usually would affect less than the entire thickness of the heart. However, non-Q-wave heart attacks are no less dangerous than the Q-wave forms. In fact, there is some evidence to suggest that the post-discharge prognosis may actually be *worse*, since the involved coronary artery is less likely to be totally occluded; cardiologists know that sooner or later it *will* become totally occluded. In other words, more trouble is on the way. "Sitting on a powder keg" is how we often refer to this situation in talking to patients.

If a heart attack is aborted by clot-busting or PTCA, the patient's stay in the hospital will be only several days to a week.

If not, and if there are no complications, the stay will be a week to ten days. Prior to going home, a low-level exercise test will be performed. This tells the physician whether residual ischemia is present; it also reassures the patient that it is OK to go home and resume normal activities without feeling the need of the hospital's support system. Often a rehabilitation program is recommended for several months, with return to work in two to three months. If the patient's course is complicated by fluid buildup, angina or irregular heartbeats, more time in the hospital may be necessary to correct the problems. For example, digitalis or diuretics (water-pills), are given for fluid buildup. For persistent angina or ischemia on the exercise test, especially after a non-Q wave heart attack, balloon angioplasty or coronary surgery may be necessary. Arrhythmias are treated with antiarrhythmic drugs.

In the final analysis, long term survival depends on how much good heart muscle remains. That is why today's cardiologist is not content to relieve pain while heart muscle dies but rather wants to save as much of the heart as possible. For this reason, cardiologists have been especially excited by the results of several trials showing that a new class of drugs (ACE-inhibitors, described earlier for blood pressure control) are also valuable in the post heart attack period. These drugs appear to help the heart in the post heart attack period by affecting "remodeling"—that is, minimize thinning of the surviving wall and keeping the heart's pumping action as effective as possible. One study in particular provided striking evidence of this approach. The Survival and Ventricular Enlargement (SAVE) trial enrolled 2231 patients who had heart attacks and weakened heart muscle but *without* overt evidence of heart failure (fluid collection in the lungs, legs, or both.) If they had heart failure, the ACE-inhibitors would certainly be indicated, but what made this study intriguing was its goal in *preventing* the development of heart failure in patients with a propensity for it due to weakened heart muscle. Patients were given either captopril or a placebo. Mortality for all cases was significantly reduced in the one year follow-up period (as reported in the *New England*

Journal of Medicine in 1992) as was the incidence of repeat heart attacks and the development of overt heart failure.

Although cardiologists obviously have a wide array of tools to help heart attack victims, one point must be emphasized. For all these drugs and procedures to work best, it is the patient who gets to the hospital early who helps the doctors save heart muscle—and, of course, the patients help themselves even more.

12

Living with Heart Disease: Psychological and Sexual Implications for Patient and Family

Living with heart disease requires changes in the lives of the patient and the family. Oftentimes the medical and nursing staffs take excellent care of the physical needs of the patient, ignoring the fact that full recovery also implies addressing the psychological needs of the family and the patient. If families are unable to return to their previous way of functioning, family, individual or group psychotherapy may be indicated.

The helicopter landing field at the State University of New York Health Sciences Center at Stony Brook is adjacent to the University Hospital. It is marked—appropriately enough— with a large red cross insignia. Many patients with heart disease are airlifted to Stony Brook from community hospitals all over central and eastern Long Island. These patients are given "high priority" during their transfer as, of course, they should be. Only later do the families arrive, in their cars or by whatever means of transport they can find.

The families of the patients come as afterthoughts to many physicians—physicians who pride themselves in providing the best possible care for their patients. Families should be more than afterthoughts. If physicians are successful and their patients live, it is the family, especially the spouse and children, that will be a major source of support during the convalescence and rehabilitation period. It is also the family that will have their own concerns (emotional, financial) with which to contend. Just as the patient has to learn to live with heart disease, so does the patient's family.

Internists and cardiologists often refer patients and/or their families to one of us (JKC) for short-term crisis intervention following the diagnosis of coronary artery disease, a heart attack, or bypass surgery. Patients and families may feel estranged from each other, not knowing what is expected of them. Living with heart disease is a particularly challenging and difficult situation for both patient and family. The heart is such a vital organ that the diagnosis that one's heart is impaired is very frightening. The language of love and caring always refers to the importance of having a "good" heart, a "loving" heart, a "healthy" heart. Thus, the heart becomes the physical and psychological symbol of life.

This chapter will help the reader understand the reactions patients have when they find out that they have heart disease, what they must do in order to live with angina or hypertension, and how they can adjust to life after having experienced a heart attack or having undergone cardiac surgery. In addition, the chapter will address the attitudes and reactions of the families of the cardiac patient. One of the questions most frequently asked is when one can resume sexual activity. People mistakenly think that sexual intercourse is more dangerous than vacuuming the house or shoveling snow.

There are many similar reactions that all cardiac patients have, but each person must be seen and evaluated as an individual. Cardiac patients will often cope with their disease in a similar manner to the way they have coped with any previous disease or adversity in their lives.

There are two extreme psychological reactions to cardiac disease, both of which can harm the individual. One occurs in patients who completely deny that there is anything wrong with them. They refuse to adhere to the medical regimen prescribed by the cardiologist. They refuse medication, continue to smoke, and do not modify their diet or exercise programs. The other occurs in patients who hear the diagnosis of heart disease and decide that the only proper and safe way to live is to pamper themselves and be pampered by others. They quit their jobs, never go out or have fun, and thus become what is known as a "cardiac cripple." In between are various ways of coping, but most important and necessary for the health of the patient and family is avoiding the extremes.

How is this done? It is our experience, and that of other health care professionals, that patients and their families need to have as full an understanding of the disease as possible. This may mean that if patients are initially unable to ask questions because they are in a state of shock, a spouse, sibling or older child may have to intervene, sit down with the doctor with pen and paper in hand and try to get a full picture of the patient's condition and regimen. Does the lifestyle need to change? Sometimes it does because of unhealthy ways of living—smoking, lack of exercise, obesity, magnitude of stress. What medication is being prescribed? What are the expected side effects? Are they harmful, etc.? How often should the patient see the doctor and what is the role of the family? The physician needs to be available for consultation for the medical needs of the patient on an ongoing basis, as well as to evaluate whether the patient and/or family can use additional help from a social worker, psychologist or psychiatrist for their psychological needs. A psychiatrist is indicated when the patient has had a previous history of emotional problems that have necessitated the use of anti-depressant or other drug therapy. Family physicians and internists who have known the family prior to the onset of the disease are in an ideal position to evaluate the family's coping skills and to decide if the family needs short-term psychotherapy.

It is important to realize that the experience of heart disease puts the patient and family in a position where they feel anxious about their future health and lifestyle. When people experience a lack of control over their lives, they often become angry and depressed. In March of 1993, Bill Moyers hosted a major series on public television illustrating the importance of the mind-body connection. He demonstrated that the psychological reaction—how patients cope with disease—impacts greatly on prognosis. The mind affects the body and its health, and the health of the body affects how one feels about oneself and one's environment. How the patient and family react psychologically often determines the outcome of the disease to a much greater degree than physicians often recognize. Sometimes a crisis situation can motivate patients and families to convert negative behavior into healthy adaptation.

The reader may get a better understanding of the psychological implications of heart disease by relating them to individual cardiac problems, by seeing how one reacts to these situations and how they should be handled ideally.

Mr. Cole comes to his internist, Dr. Bowen, because he has experienced a peculiar pain in his right arm that seems to be affecting his jaws and gums. Mr. Cole is a stockbrocker who each day works for 12 hours, smokes two packs of cigarettes, and commutes a minimum of two hours to his office. At age 50, he is 6 feet tall and weighs 235 pounds. His eating is somewhat erratic and irregular, but usually he has two eggs, a serving of bacon or sausage, three pieces of toast with extra butter, and coffee with cream and sugar for breakfast with similar excesses at later meals. For example, at night Mrs. Cole usually makes roast beef, steak, lamb, or beef stew interspersed with an occasional creamed chicken or fish followed by dessert.

Let us see how Mr. Cole reacts when Dr. Bowen informs him that he, indeed, has angina. There is no reason for Mr. Cole to panic. Although Dr. Bowen encourages him to continue to enjoy his life, he also stresses that Mr. Cole does need to change his lifestyle in order to treat his coronary artery disease.

Mr. Cole is told that many things he is presently doing are hazardous to his health. Perhaps most evident is his consumption of between two and four packs of cigarettes per day. These have got to go! The physician gives him helpful hints to make the process easier (see Chapter 7). It is difficult to quit, but for the cardiac patient it is essential. People often think that smoking is something they cannot live without, but in fact it's something they cannot live with.

Mr. Cole also needs to lose weight and change his eating patterns. People often ask how they can do both, especially at the same time. It can be done, perhaps with difficulty, but if Mr. Cole is willing and determined to protect his heart, he can succeed. Actually, it may be easier to change both diet and smoking regimens at the same time. Two of the most important aspects of breaking any habit are (1) wanting to break it and (2) changing the routine that triggers the brain. For example, Mr. Cole drinks an enormous amount of coffee with cream. Excessive caffeine and any cream are not good for his condition. When he drinks this concoction, it stimulates his brain, and he reaches for a cigarette—that is, he associates drinking coffee with smoking cigarettes. Mr. Cole should stop putting cream in his coffee (skimmed milk or nothing would be far better), which would probably cut down his consumption of coffee. If he could, switching to moderate amounts of coffee or tea (less than three cups per day) or consuming fluids that don't have caffeine would be sensible alternatives. Thus, Mr. Cole would be drinking something—not coffee—that will cut down or eliminate the cream, the caffeine and the association between coffee and cigarettes.

Dr. Bowen also suggests a change of diet. Mr. Cole is consuming large amounts of food that contain cholesterol. As we noted in Chapter 8, in August 1986 the American Heart Association recommended that a person's total intake of fat be limited to less than 30% of all caloric intake. The Association indicated that saturated fat be reduced to less than 10% of all caloric intake, with the rest made up of polyunsaturated fat. Cholesterol intake should not be more than 300 mg per day. The new guidelines also recommended consuming not more than 1 teaspoon (3g) of salt per day. People who drink should limit themselves to no more than 1.5 ounces of alcohol (two mixed drinks, 24 ounces of beer or two 4-ounce glasses of wine). This means that Mr. Cole must not eat eggs and butter daily, should consume beef and lamb only occasionally and should change his diet to include chicken, fish, vegetable and pasta dishes that are not smothered in cream (see Chapter 8).

LIVING WITH ANGINA

What else should the patient be doing in order to live successfully with angina? One of the most important aspects of living with angina is becoming tuned in to your body. One should get immediate help if the pattern of the angina changes. These changes may manifest themselves in different ways. Angina should be brought to your doctor's attention when it:

1. Occurs more often.
2. Occurs even though you haven't had a lot of activity.
3. Lasts longer.
4. Isn't relieved by your medication.
5. Occurs at a time that is unusual for you.
6. Seems more frequent or much more severe than usual.

We have thus far portrayed Mr. Cole as the ideal patient: the patient who is ready, willing, and able to change his lifestyle in order to prolong his life. Unfortunately, there are other patients who do not react as rationally to the diagnosis of heart disease.

No one wants to be sick, especially with heart disease — which kills more people each year than any other disease, more than cancer and AIDS combined. Mr. Knight has also been to see Dr. Bowen because of "just not feeling right" and has also been diagnosed as having heart disease. His pain has been mostly in his jaws and teeth, and he has experienced shortness of breath. However, Mr. Knight has a different reaction to the diagnosis. He becomes very hostile and angry with Dr. Bowen, calls him ignorant and stupid, and questions his abilities as a doctor. After his abusive outburst, Mr. Knight leaves the office. Two days later he experiences a choking sensation combined with shortness of breath and becomes very frightened. He goes to see another internist, gets the same diagnosis of angina pectoris, and calls Dr. Bowen again.

Dr. Bowen prescribes a similar regimen for Mr. Knight as he did for Mr. Cole, including a change of diet, exercise, and stress-related activities. Mr. Knight shows his disbelief and anger in a rather exaggerated way, but, in fact, this happens quite frequently. Because heart disease implies a loss of health, similar to a loss via death, patients may proceed through the stages that Dr. Elisabeth Kubler-Ross describes in those people facing knowledge of terminal illness or death: denial, anger, bargaining, acceptance and hope.

Mr. Knight becomes the perfect patient for about a month, by losing about 5 pounds and stopping smoking. He tells Dr. Bowen that he will do everything the doctor said as long as he feels fine and can return to his previous lifestyle. However, after a month of abstinence, smoking and eating excessively—as well as 12-hour days at the office—resume. This behavior is halted only when he has a heart attack and is hospitalized. We will see Mr. Knight again later in this chapter.

A third patient, Mr. Fiore, is diagnosed with coronary artery disease after coming to Dr. Bowen with symptoms of extreme tiredness and a constant burning, squeezing pressure in the upper stomach. Mr. Fiore has a different reaction to the diagnosis than either Mr. Cole or Mr. Knight. When he leaves Dr. Bowen's office, he throws away his pack of cigarettes, eats no meat or cheese, and asks for a change of job to a passive, less demanding position—even though he has to accept a cut in salary. In addition, he refuses to go outside and play ball with his children and will not go out on weekend evenings with his wife. Each weekend afternoon, he takes a two-hour nap. Mr. Fiore has assumed the role of a cardiac cripple, a person who is afraid he can do nothing because he has heart disease.

We have described three men in their early 50s who have worked at high-pressure, demanding jobs that produced great feelings of stress. Stress may have contributed to their over-weight, smoking, lack of exercise, and generally unhealthful habits. Since they appear to be so similar, how does one account for the different reaction to the doctor's diagnosis of heart disease in these patients? The way in which the doctor presents the diagnosis to the patient affects the situation a great deal. Is it presented in a matter-of-fact manner? Or is there too much negative information and not enough encouragement? A crisis situation is created when people find that their life span may be shortened because their heart is not functioning properly. People's reactions to crises are based on many different things. Perhaps most important is the manner in which a successful resolution of crises has been achieved in the past. If a patient has a history of mental illness and inappropriate or exaggerated reactions to crises in the past, adjusting to the diagnosis may be difficult and a mental health professional should be available for consultation by the patient and/or family. If, however, patients are surrounded by a caring, supportive system that reacts without panic, that system will give them the kind of additional strength necessary to begin to cope.

The knowledge that one has coronary artery disease and could be headed for an untimely death causes anxiety and fear in everyone. This is understandable, since there is lack of knowledge as to whether one may suffer a heart attack and death, or whether the disease will linger, hardly affecting the patient. A relationship of trust needs to be developed between the patient and the doctor. Sometimes patients refuse to follow the advice of their physician merely because they feel misunderstood or ignored. Many doctors schedule their patients' visits too close together to be able to address the individual needs of the patient and family. If patients are truly unable to trust, respect and talk with their doctor, then a change of doctor may be appropriate.

What about the physician's point of view? One patient listens to medical advice and is appreciative of the physician's expertise; another patient is hostile and angry and questions the doctor's abilities as a person, as well as a medical professional.

The practice may be so active that the physician does not have the time necessary to address the emotional needs of all patients. In addition, many physicians do not have the training to understand the psychological ramifications of having a life-threatening disease. We would suggest that physicians who cannot or will not make time to address these needs should have a nurse practictioner in the office to fill in medical information and give emotional support. A social worker, psychologist or psychiatrist should be available as a mental health consultant for emotional problems brought on or exaggerated by the diagnosis of heart disease.

The three patients we described, who were diagnosed with coronary artery disease accompanied by painful symptoms, exhibited three rather typical ways of coping with the news. Mr. Cole did things right. He realized that the doctor's diagnosis necessitated caution and a need for change in his lifestyle and diet. However, he didn't panic and feel that a change would mean disaster. His attitude toward life seems to be if change is required, then he will find a way to do it!

Mr. Knight, however, denied that anything could happen to him. He felt that he was in his 50s, the prime of his life, enjoying the financial rewards of middle age. He was unwilling and/or unable to recognize that anger, denial and "bargaining" with his doctor could not ameliorate his cardiac condition. Unfortunately, denial is a common way of dealing with heart disease. One afternoon one of us (JKC) was seeing a couple in marital therapy when the man started rubbing his arm. He said that he had just taken up tennis because he had gained some additional weight. His wife said that she had been urging him to check out what was wrong with his arm, but he had refused. JKC interceded and suggested he follow through with his wife's request. He went to his internist that afternoon and was sent to a cardiologist the same day. The electrocardiogram showed an abnormality. Three weeks later he underwent triple-bypass surgery. This man had been denying his pain, hoping that it did not indicate heart disease. We sometimes wonder what would have happened to him if he hadn't come for therapy that day or hadn't been willing to listen to advice!

Our third patient, Mr. Fiore, panicked. Heart disease, for whatever reason, connoted death. Everything in his life seemed to have to change in order for him to continue living. He needed to realize that one does not have to become a cardiac cripple in order to live a long life.

The reaction of the patient's family to the diagnosis is often the most important element in how well the patient copes with his or her disease. Spouses and children provide the core of emotional support that a patient may need to face news that can be earth-shattering. Numerous studies have shown that patients recover and function at a higher level when they have a good supportive network.

INDIVIDUAL FAMILY MEMBERS' REACTION TO HEART DISEASE

All members of the family have different reactions to the patient's illness, based on their relationship to the patient and their individual developmental stage and their own coping skills. The case histories below illustrate this point.

Mrs. Wallace, age 73, has been diagnosed as having coronary artery disease. Her husband had a heart attack last year and died. She is presently living near her only son's family. Her son, David, has two boys, ages 15 and 11. David, age 40, had the misfortune of having had two contemporaries at his brokerage office have heart attacks within the last year.

David Wallace had never really thought about heart disease until his father died. He had read about the need for people to modify their lifestyles but felt that the warnings really didn't pertain to him. When his mother's doctor called to tell him that she would need help running her home, a crisis looms on the horizon. Her illness will affect all aspects of David's life. He realizes that he might not get a housekeeper to take care of his mother, so perhaps she will have to move in with his family. How will this affect his wife and sons? Because he has been surrounded by so many people being stricken with heart disease, he decides that he will go in for a checkup. At that time, the doctor tells David that because his uncle (and probably his father) had coronary artery disease while they were young, he had better re-evaluate his own situation. His cigarette smoking and "devil-may-care" attitude toward food will have to go. All of a sudden David becomes laden with a sick mother, the knowledge that he has three risk factors for heart disease and the fear that he will suffer the same fate as his friends and family.

The family of Arthur Kraft also faces problems when Arthur has a heart attack. Arthur, age 41, is a corporate attorney. He has three children, Michelle, 15, Jonathan, 10, and Ari, 5. The children are all very upset because they assumed they caused the attack by aggravating their father the night before he became ill. Michelle had wanted to go to a friend's party when the parents weren't at home; father had been vehement about her not going. The argument that followed had been Michelle's last interaction with her father before his attack. Jonathan had insisted that Arthur help his friends prepare their equipment for their Boy Scout outing, even though his father had insisted that he was too tired and had an important brief to review before an upcoming trial. That was Jonathan's last conversation with his father before the attack. Ari had told his dad that he hated him because he wanted to sit on his mother's lap at the dinner table, and Dad had emphatically said no. Thus, each child had aggravated Mr. Kraft shortly before he went to bed the night preceeding his heart attack. Their behavior was absolutely normal, childlike behavior—yet they felt guilty and scared that their actions had caused their father's illness.

When an illness, accident or death occurs without prior warning, family members are afraid that their negative interaction with the afflicted person has caused the situation. It is important to dispel this idea as quickly as possible, especially with children. Encourage children to talk about their guilt feelings, as well as their own fear of dying—feelings that often accompany the heart attack of a parent.

Both families need to evaluate their eating habits as well. Because relatives had heart attacks at such an early age, the children may eventually be at risk as well. Heart-healthy eating is important for all families, but it is essential for those who have a parent who has had heart disease at an early age. It would be most helpful to change the diet gradually (over a month or so) to prevent the children from having a need to act out and disobey their parents because they feel frustrated and deprived by the new regimen.

Miriam Stark, 39, is among a small percentage of women who have heart attacks before menopause. Mrs. Stark has elevated cholesterol levels, is a cigarette smoker and has taken birth-control pills for the past twelve years. These three factors increase the likelihood that premenopausal women will develop heart disease. Mrs. Stark works at home as a mother, housekeeper and wife. Her responsibilities include child care, carpooling, grocery shopping, cooking, and clothes shopping—which represent the workloads of a nurse, party planner, chauffeur, at-home teacher, clothes consultant, etc. Instead of the breadwinner being the patient, it is now the "bread baker" who is the patient. Her husband is a corporate executive who has always left the care of the house and family to "the little woman." Now this family must adjust to not having available the "Jill of All Trades and Mistress of Everything!"

Spouses of heart patients, whether they be male or female, have to re-adjust their lives and take on new and additional responsibilities. Mr. Stark had been used to his wife handling all his domestic needs and those of his children. Now he will either have to change his lifestyle or hire people to help him take care of his family. He feels overwhelmed by the changes in his life. He can barely take care of his own needs (such as picking up his laundry), much less arrange for housecleaning, cooking, carpooling for the children, etc. When the children express a fear of impending death of their mother and themselves, he is unable to help them.

Immediately following a crisis—such as a parent having a heart attack—children need a sympathetic ear, preferably from their healthy parent. This is also not a good time to make major lifestyle changes that might result in children feeling insecure and deprived. It is important for the patient, as well as the children, that the home assumes a normal posture as soon as possible following the crisis. One of JKC's female patients had a father with chronic heart disease. She was not allowed to go on school trips, to school proms or out with her friends. Instead of going out and playing, she had the responsibility of taking care of her father after school and on weekends. She never had a normal childhood and felt old before her time. Consequently, when she married and had a child, she felt overwhelmed by the change in her lifestyle and the additional responsibility demanded by her infant son. In her mind, she equated her son with her father, although the situations were dissimilar. The needs of her father should not have been thrust on her young shoulders.

LIVING WITH SILENT HEART DISEASE

Silent coronary artery disease presents a more complicated picture for the physician, the patient and the family. As we have seen, the patient has no pain but can have the same amount of disease, which can result in sudden death. Naturally, the patient who is diagnosed as having silent heart disease has the same fears and anxieties as the patient with angina, but it is much easier to deny the disease component because one may feel fine and have no symptoms. Many people are angry that they are deprived of a proper warning system to help regulate their lifestyles. As one would suspect, our research has shown that the patient with silent disease shows a greater degree of surprise at the diagnosis than does the patient with painful angina. We also have found that patients often feel a need to do something "different" with their lifestyles, in the hope that this change will arrest the course of the disease. This desire has sometimes had paradoxical results: Those who had exercised before stop their exercise, and those who had led sedentary lives begin to exercise.

The physician must realize that the patient and the family of a patient with silent coronary artery disease may need special time and attention and must be aware of how the patient and family are coping. The physician should also determine whether the patient's and family's reactions to the diagnosis are within a normal range; if not, individual or family counseling should be recommended. The way in which disease is handled by spouse and children often reflects how the family functions, as well as the psychopathology in the family.

The fact that the life-threatening disease is silent may cause more problems than when a disease is apparent through discomfort or pain. The patient may have more difficulty modulating self-indulgent and self-destructive behavior when he or she feels perfectly fine. A marathon runner who had silent ischemia needed extra time and understanding from PFC to make him realize that he might be able to resume his activities after evaluation and treatment, but that until then continuing to run such distances was foolhardly and downright dangerous.

As with the patient with angina, the family's reaction to the disease greatly affects the patient. The family needs to understand how asymptomatic disease is different from, as well as similar to, painful coronary artery disease. Patients must achieve a delicate balance between living a normal lifestyle and knowing when they need to avoid situations in which they are over-stressed or overexerted. Patients report that their families are hard-pressed to change long-held expectations; laundry should be done, garbage and snow removal should be executed pronto! A hard concept for both the patient and family to accept is that one has to moderate or cease an activity despite the lack of symptoms.

LIVING WITH A HEART ATTACK

The interaction between the patient, the doctor and the family becomes very intricate and complicated when the cardiac patient has suffered a heart attack.

As we have emphasized, people often deny that they are having angina or unusual feelings that they may have never felt before. Similarly, we hear patients say after they have had a heart attack that they thought they were just having indigestion—although it really didn't feel as if food had caused the discomfort. The denial of symptoms that prevents the patient from going immediately to the emergency room of the local hospital may hinder full recovery and even result in death. Current studies indicate that the median time of delay ranges from three to five hours. One may say, so what? But 55–80% of deaths that result from heart attacks occur within four hours of the beginning of the attack. If many people did not pretend the discomfort was not related to heart disease, their lives could have been saved. In addition, new techniques like thrombolysis and angioplasty (described in Chapter 11) can be used to minimize whatever damage might have occurred during the heart attack.

Why do people not move quickly and get to the hospital as soon as possible? People deny that bad things are happening to them when they are fearful or feel in personal danger. ("This could never happen to me.") They think the pain is due to indigestion or muscle aches—perhaps from having played too much racketball over the weekend! People also feel that they are too young; only the elderly have heart conditions. Chest pain may signify to otherwise healthy adults that their life is over, their future will be horrible or they will be marred for life. These are all not true. Many patients survive a heart attack, can return to work and can have a basically similar lifestyle to the one they had previously. Some patients, however, risk becoming an invalid after a heart attack because they have denied the symptoms for so long that, by the time they receive medical attention, they have unnecessarily jeopardized both their lifestyle and their life. One must either act on one's own or, if necessary, be brought under protest to the hospital if symptoms do occur. Better to incur the wrath of a friend or family member than have him permanently injured or dead!

Patients who have had a heart attack may feel a loss of control over themselves and their lives. Often heart attacks come without previous recognizable cardiac symptoms and patients are caught unaware. Family members, friends and business associates may have feelings of guilt because of some extra stressful events they may have caused. In this way, the heart attack creates fear, anxiety and uncertainty for patient and family and thus a crisis is at hand. Thus, prior methods of functioning both physically and emotionally may no longer be valid.

Naturally, the patient and family have very different experiences during the initial period following the heart attack and during recovery while in the hospital. For example, when the patient is brought to the emergency room of a hospital complaining of pain that appears to be from the heart, there is often much hustle and bustle—as exemplified by the scene described at the beginning of the chapter. It is important to re-emphasize that patients are often not told in detail about essential tests that are being administered. They should be provided with knowledge of what is happening to them and what the medical facts are. Their questions should be answered with as much honesty and reassurance as possible. Dr. B. Cowie suggests that the patient needs to understand the factors that contributed to the illness. By constructing a series of circumstances and events, the attack will make more sense, thus eliminating many intense childlike, fearful feelings. Patients should be told in the most optimistic fashion just what has happened and what the future might hold. They are better off hearing the truth. If the patient is somehow aware of deceit, the necessary trustful relationship between patient and doctor never develops.

A study reported by Dr. R. Klein and associates at the University of North Carolina in 1965 suggests that patients who act as if they are invalids after having had a heart attack do so as a result of the initial interactions between the physician, patient and family. In other words, the patient became confused because he was not given the necessary information to understand just what has happened, or the information was given in an insensitive way. It is important for the patient to have this knowledge and assimilate it to proceed along the road to a full recovery.

Even when medical procedures in a hospital are being performed well, patients' families may be ignored and even at times insulted by hospital staff. Because a family member—often the father—has been affected, the homeostasis of the family changes.

Someone must fill the various gaps that are left by the heart attack victim. It is essential that the medical staff take time to fully inform the family about the patient's attack and expected recovery routine while in the hospital. Family members will then be able to compensate for the loss of the patient in the day-to-day functioning of the family.

After a brief stay in the emergency ward, a patient is usually transferred to the coronary care unit. The stay there can last from several days to several weeks, depending on the patient's condition and the progress of the recovery period. During that time, the patient has almost no contact with anyone other than fellow patients and medical staff. Immediate members of the family are allowed to visit, and only for a few minutes at a time. Once again, the patient should be informed about the nature of his or her illness using tact, discretion and reassurance. When a patient feels that information is being hidden, it not only destroys the trust in others, but he or she may experience a fantasy of imminent death—they're only telling me a little or keeping secrets from me; therefore, I must be very sick and about to die.

It is also imperative that procedures and medications be explained to the patient; why they are being administered and what side effects, if any, might occur as a result. Naturally, patients will be fearful in such a highly technical, unusual, and ominous environment; they will feel anxiety and should be encouraged to talk about it. They often wonder if they will survive. Alarms on the electrocardiogram contribute to the anxiety. They may indicate an emergency for the patient or for someone else—or may have been set off by mistake!

Thus fear, anxiety and depression are normal and expected reactions to the situation. However, if the anxiety level prevents the patient from getting the needed rest essential for a healthy recovery, specific medication and/or a mental health consultation may be indicated.Often it is helpful for a nurse, social worker, psychologist or psychiatrist to speak with the patient to clarify the nature and source of the feelings of anxiety. (In extreme cases, a panic attack can be treated by the cardiologist and psychiatrist together.) It is important to remember that these psychological situations are almost always temporary and short-lived; they are normal reactions to a life-threatening situation. By being honest and open with patients, negative psychological reactions can frequently be minimized.

When family members enter the CCU to visit the patient, they may feel overwhelmed. The CCU is a small space filled with the sights, smells and sounds of illness. One finds odors of medication, unusual sights of high-tech instruments and the deep sighs and moans of the troubled breathing of the patients. The patients often look dreadful because their bodies have undergone a severe shock. Also, they may look drugged and talk in an unintelligible way. The family may find the patient disoriented because of the effects of the heart attack and because the world of the CCU is very insulated and protective. Patients receive little mental or emotional stimulation. Families of patients may experience the same anxiety, fear and depression as the patient does. Spouses and children experience great uncertainty as to how this crisis will affect them directly. In what way will their lifestyles have to change?

It is essential to the well-being of the patient that the family be included in the treatment plan. Just as in the emergency room setting, families need to know what is going on in the CCU, what the prognosis is and what to expect physically and psychologically from the patient during the stay in the unit. Too often, families are shunted aside so that they are unaware of what is happening. In some CCUs the staff considers the family a potentially disruptive influence and controls their behavior by excluding them. Families feel that the medical and nursing staff gives them little or no time to discuss the patient's prognosis, thus offering no emotional or psychological support. Research indicates time and time again that recovery from illness is dependent not only on the physical and emotional condition of the patient but on the family's response, support and understanding as well. In addition to a meeting with the cardiologist, it is often helpful for the family to have a meeting with a mental health professional who is knowledgeable about heart disease. This can give the family the opportunity to ask any additional questions that they might have concerning the health of the patient and its effect on family functioning. Many CCUs—in both teaching hospitals and community hospitals—are now aware of these problems and make conscious efforts to keep families apprised of the situation.

Other issues in patient–family relationships also surface during the time that the patients are in the coronary care unit, and are living in a completely different world from that of their families. The patient is being shielded from physical and emotional stress; the family is picking up the pieces that are the outcome of this crisis. The patient is resting as much as possible; the family may be frenetic, trying to fit those precious moments of visiting into a busy schedule. The patient is encouraged to begin moving about as soon as possible; the family may react with trepidation that something harmful will happen, especially if they are ignorant of normal hospital procedures. These disparate experiences can create tension that needs to be diffused.

When patients are moved from the coronary care unit to a bed in a regular hospital room, a new set of reactions can occur. Although they have gradually started to walk about and exercise, being reassured that these steps forward lead to recovery, leaving the coronary care unit means leaving the security of monitors and the intensive nursing care. Although the CCU machines may have initially been frightening, they later provided reassurance. However uneasy the patient may feel leaving the CCU, the family is often more displeased and worried. This is a stage during which the patient and family must come together and achieve a balance after having been separated for days or weeks. The family may impede the recovery of the patient by overprotection, which can result from being unaware about what activities have been encouraged by the medical staff to build confidence, strength and endurance. It is important for both patient and family to once again be informed by the medical staff as to what is indicated for the patient's recovery, so that additional tension is not created by differing expectations or lack of knowledge. Patients are used to following the advice of the medical personnel rather than the family. The patient may be encouraged to do more and more, and this positive movement forward can be thwarted by the attitude of the family. If the situation indeed becomes problematic and cannot be handled by the family, a mental health practitioner's intervention, especially one skilled in family dynamics, would be a great help to all concerned (patient, medical staff and family).

Of the thousands of people who survive heart attacks each year and are physically able to resume normal lives by returning to previous work and leisure time activities, many do not because of psychological reasons. Dr. Mark A. Hlatky and colleagues from Duke University reported in 1986 that poor patient adjustment following a heart attack, rather than heart damage itself, affected whether or not the patients saw themselves as disabled indefinitely. People who were depressed or thought that they were more ill than they actually were, were more likely not to return to work—regardless of their medical condition. The most important prognosticator of how well patients will recover from a heart attack is the emotional makeup of both patient and family, which affects how well he or she will adjust to living with the disease. Often the patients become depressed as a reaction to the loss of good health, viewing themselves as defective.

During the first week of convalescence at home following a heart attack, patients often will feel physically weak just by exerting themselves a little. The patient has been insulated in the hospital, where all care, and responsibility has been in the hands of others. The re-entrance into the family and the reality of life can indeed be traumatic. Patients may be gloomy, prone to tears and feel life is hopeless. They may also suffer from anorexia (no desire to eat), become apathetic and take little pleasure in interaction with the environment, thus experiencing an even greater sense of loss and isolation. Some people may become suicidal. Care should be taken by the physician and family to assess how active the suicidal plans may be. If patients voice no hope in the future and speak of ending their life to their family, the family should consult the cardiologist immediately. Depression can be brought on or aggravated by drugs being used to treat the cardiac condition. Anti-depressants may be indicated. The prescribing physician must know the possible side effects of such drugs (especially when they interact with cardiovascular drugs) and treat the patient accordingly.

If the patient does not respond to changing the cardiac medication or introduction of anti-depressants, referral to a psychiatrist should be considered. When the patient and/or family requests help, or if there are problems within the family, a referral to a social worker, psychologist or psychiatrist for individual, marital or family therapy would be advisable. If the person suffers from chest pain and/or arrhythmias, the feelings of depression and hopelessness can return. This can be attributed to the fact that the person has a constant reminder of ill health. Patients no longer believe that they will live forever and feel vulnerable to another heart attack.

Usually the depression lifts within the first month following the heart attack, as the person resumes some normal activities such as seeing friends and family. Remember that just the resumption of talking and being social can be difficult for a person who has been secluded within the hospital setting. Making small gains (for example, climbing steps or going for a walk) gives the patient confidence that a normal lifestyle is possible.

Any patient who is able to perform everyday activities without cardio-respiratory discomfort can resume sexual activity without any cause for concern. The resumption of sexual intercourse is an important event for the cardiac patient's ego. The patient experiences love and intimacy at the same time as feeling strong physically. Resumption of sexual activity helps to solidify the marital relationship during a stressful period. It is a myth that cardiac patients often die during intercourse, at the precise moment of orgasm. Actually, most reported deaths during sexual intercourse (which are uncommon) occur when the partner is someone other than the spouse. One suspects that the cause of the person's demise could be related to stress or anxiety over adultery rather than the act itself. If patients have no symptoms during regular daily activity and have the desire and capability to initiate sexual intercourse, they will usually have no complications during or after the sexual act. The reality is that many everyday tasks require much more oxygen intake than does intercourse!

Patients are often uncomfortable about taking the cardiologist's time to talk about their sexual needs, but it is important for each patient to consult his or her own physician to be sure that there is no contra-indication to resume sexual intercourse. This is usually appropriate at the four week checkup after the heart attack at which time an exercise test is often recommended. If the checkup is normal, the physician will suggest resumption of daily activities, including sexual intercourse. We explain to patients that any sexual activity they desire can be started as long as their post-heart attack course is proceeding satisfactorily. Some couples may feel more secure by initially having a sexual relationship based on less active participation by the affected partner. For example, couples often feel more relaxed when the afflicted spouse occupies the lower, passive position beneath his or her mate. Alternatively, the unaffected spouse may stimulate the affected partner through oral sex, other forms of foreplay or masturbation. After the cardiac patient has had orgasms without incident, the couple may be ready for a more physically active sexual relationship. Sexual intercourse is an important component of the recovery period.

In most cases, whatever the sexual relationship between patient and spouse was prior to the heart attack will be the optimum level of activity after the attack. In most cases, the patient and spouse will not have a more active sex life than before the heart attack. However, if a couple had intimacy problems before the heart attack, the fear of losing one another may motive them to have a more active sexual life.

Another important part of the recovery period for many patients is their participation in a cardiac rehabilitation program. Most hospitals have access to such a program, if they do not have one of their own. There are many different kinds of cardiac rehabilitation programs, but they all have the aim of returning patients to their physical, psychological and social conditions prior to the heart attack.

Participation in a cardiac rehabilitation program provides a necessary support system for the patient. Often, when a person has a heart attack, they have a loss of self-esteem, as well as an inordinate fear that the previous lifestyle cannot be resumed. A person who is involved in a group rehabilitation program more often achieves restoration of previous physical and emotional strength. Cardiac rehabilitation programs usually have two components: one for physical therapy and support and one to improve the emotional well-being of the patient. The patient is expected to participate regularly in an exercise program and, in some programs, to be part of a psychotherapeutic support group. It is within this context that many patients have found the strength to give up smoking and initiate a regular exercise program on their own. The exercise program is individually designed for the patient and includes activities such as walking, swimming and biking (see Chapter 9). This increased sense of control and "doing something for oneself" leads to a greater sense of self-esteem that counteracts the loss of confidence resulting from having been a victim of a heart attack.

Psychological cardiac rehabilitation groups start while the patient is still in the hospital. These groups include the patients and/or their spouses and provide a forum for airing questions, concerns and anxieties about the patient's and the family's future. Just what is permissible and advisable when I leave the hospital? How does the heart work and why and how do heart attacks occur? How can I delete or decrease the stress from my life and adjust to my new life now? How often can I go out with my spouse on weekends? What games can I play with my children? Including the spouse in some aspects of the process helps to educate the family and encourage compliance.

Drs. R. Erdman and H. Duivenoorden from Duke University reported in a 1983 study of 64 patients that those who participated in a structured rehabilitation program functioned better psychologically (less depression, etc.) than those who did not. It is within this context that patients develop new friends who have had similar experiences and are thus capable of understanding them more fully.

RECOVERY FROM CORONARY BYPASS SURGERY

Several studies have shown that surgically treated heart patients were significantly less depressed than those patients treated medically. They also report not only that they feel better, but that their families seem to function better as well.

Why is this true? Medical treatment often involves complicated drug therapy that requires the patient to take the prescribed medicines and to keep in close contact with the physician for checkups. The use of heart drugs may involve a complex "try one and change" routine on the part of the physician. Physicians must be well versed in the many drugs available, as well as their side effects and complications, especially when they are to be used in tandem with other drugs. Trials of different medical regimens require fortitude, understanding, and tolerance from both the patient and the physician.

On the other hand, surgery is a dramatic event that can provide remarkable changes in overall activity within a short period of time. Surgery provides a type of instant gratification. It is as if the responsibility for feeling better is put in someone else's hands—the surgeon's. People who are debilitated by heart disease often want someone to take over their care, just as their parents did when they were children. They feel they can count on the skill of the surgeon and surgical team to make them all better.

Nevertheless, recovery from surgery is not without its problems. The physical strain can be considerable. The patient is in a surgical intensive care unit for several days after the operation, or longer if there are complications. In addition to the intravenous tubes, there are also drainage tubes from the chest for a day or two and there is usually a breathing tube which prevents talking. This is not only frightening to the patient but to the family that comes to visit, however briefly. But these problems are over when the patient leaves the surgical intensive care unit for a regular floor. All that is left are the surgical scars: the long one down the center of the chest and the smaller ones where the various tubes were inserted.

There may also be psychological scars. Although patients have been "rehabilitated" by bypass surgery and their cardiac capacities are greatly improved, many seem to lack the skills to improve their quality of life. Most people who did not work because of illness before surgery do not return to work, while those who did work pre-operatively are more likely to resume work. Thus, Dr. Hlatky's 1986 study, and others, have indicated that bypass surgery was not successful in increasing the rate of employment of patients with coronary artery disease. If a patient is well enough to work but doesn't, it is important to determine whether he or she is depressed or anxious and ameliorate that condition.

Why is it that patients who are better physically still see themselves as defective or unable to have a full, enjoyable life? Those people who have worked in boring jobs and have adequate disability insurance may not feel motivated to work again. Often patients are unaware that they are physically able to work and thus still see themselves as crippled. Just as in the emergency room and the CCU, it is very important that the physician tell both the patient and family what type of lifestyle is realistic to expect in the future. The family must be included in these discussions. Because they are often responsible for the care of the patient, their help and compliance may determine the success or failure of the rehabiliation. Each family member is affected by the loss of the role previously held by the cardiac victim. Therefore, the family as a whole has to change in order to let the person function as a strong contributing member rather than a cardiac cripple. For the male patient, if the children have left home, and the wife is retired or not working, it may be easier for the post-operative patient to remain needy just as he did before the surgery. If he is well and can take care of himself, then his wife will have to find something else to keep her occupied and fulfilled.

Psychological and physical rehabilitation of the patient after surgery is very important. It is not that dissimilar from rehabilitations after a heart attack except for being more upbeat because of the more positive attitude that things can be better now. It is helpful for the patient to be a part of a group that exercises together because such a group can become a supportive network that helps the process of recovery. People are better motivated to exercise and heed the advice of the physician and other health care professionals when they are involved in a group program. This is important because good health habits *must* continue in order to prevent a return of angina or other symptoms.

There are many psychologically oriented supportive networks, such as "Zipper Clubs,"* that are formed by a group of patients who have all undergone cardiac surgery. The group situation provides a forum for the patient to find other people who have or are experiencing similar situations and feelings as a result of the cardiac disease and its surgical treatment. These clubs become a social network for the patient, spouse and family to find kindred spirits who have experienced a similar and dramatic event. It is often helpful for the patient to have new friends who didn't know him or her "way back when."

There is every reason for the person who has undergone cardiac surgery to be optimistic about the future. Nevertheless, there are many people who remain depressed, angry and anxious. Six months after surgery, those people who are still unable to function psychologically as well as—or better than—they did pre-operatively should seek help from a social worker, psychologist or psychiatrist. Psychotherapy with patient and family— which may not need to be long-term—may provide the impetus for the patient to have a satisfying future. Sometimes we receive requests for referrals for psychotherapy years after cardiac surgery has been performed. Although the patient is now back at work and participating in physical sports, relationships with loved ones have never been restored to their pre-cardiac disease level.

---

*So-named because the scar down the middle of the chest resembles a zipper.

As noted in this chapter, the psychological ramifications of heart disease are important for the physician, patient and family. By keeping the avenues of communication open, each member of the triad can contribute to the full recovery of the cardiac patient.

CHAPTER
—— 13 ——

Women and
Heart Disease

Probably no one medical issue has captured the attention of the American public more in the last five years than the apparent inequities between attention paid to women's health issues compared to those of men. First and foremost is the concern with breast cancer. Statistics indicate that anywhere from 1 in 8 to 1 in 20 women will contract breast cancer during their lifetime; that "cure" rates have not dramatically improved in the last decade; and that even measures to reconstruct breast tissue (i.e., silicone implants) can be dangerous. Women ask, and rightly so, if the medical "establishment" would be as blasé if a similar problem of this magnitude affected a specifically male organ, like the testicles. While we in no way wish to minimize the problem of breast cancer, we feel that it is unfortunate that lost in the anger over the breast cancer problem—at least until the last several years—has been another problem: that of women's unequal treatment with regard to heart disease. Often, when women presented in a doctor's office with chest pain, their physicians would attribute their discomfort to hysteria or anxiety. Based on the fact that women who are premenopausal don't usually have heart disease, they would prescribe psychotropic medication and send them on their way. This action would make the women feel as if the doctor thought they were making up their illness and complaining. There is now ample evidence that women 1. undergo fewer diagnostic tests than men when they have chest pain complaints, and 2. even when heart disease is present, women are not treated as aggressively as men. What makes this latter controversy even more upsetting is that in terms of sheer numbers, many, many more women will die of heart disease than of breast cancer.

What is the evidence supporting these contentions? Several recent studies make the point emphatically; so much so that Dr. Bernadine Healy, a cardiologist and former Director of the National Institutes of Health, launched a crusade to increase research into both heart disease in women and the answers of the medical establishment regarding the inequity of diagnosis and care. In an editorial published in 1991 in the *New England Journal of Medicine*, she commented on two articles about gender differences in treating heart disease. Dr. Healy noted the prevalence of the diagnostic and management inequities and called for specific steps to redress these problems. She titled the article The Yentl Syndrome after the heroine of Isaac Bashevis Singer's short story about a woman who had to disguise herself as a man to gain recognition as a Talmudic scholar. The two articles that stimulated Dr. Healy's comments dealt with differences in the use of diagnostic and therapeutic procedures for coronary disease between men and women. But these were not the only such studies, nor were the conclusions necessarily the same. In a large retrospective series published in the *Annals of Internal Medicine* in 1992, the authors wondered if men were receiving an inappropriately large number of procedures rather than women receiving an inappropriately small number. At the present time, however, this represents a minority opinion.

Heart disease in women *does* present special problems, and to better understand these problems, it is best to start at the beginning. There is no question that the incidence of heart disease in women is very low in the pre-menopausal years, except in those women who have juvenile-onset diabetes, familial high cholesterol levels, or have had surgical removal of their ovaries. What is it about the female hormones that creates protection? This is not clear. Several theories have emerged, but the most popular is based on the observation that blood levels of HDL cholesterol—the "good" cholesterol—are higher in women than men but progressively decrease after the menopause when the ovaries are no longer a functioning organ providing hormones. Recent observations from Finland (also published in 1992) linking lower blood iron levels to protection from heart disease are intriguing, since women also have lower blood iron levels than men as a result of their menstrual periods. The idea that the protection afforded by female hormones is a combination of higher HDL levels and lower iron levels is an intriguing possibility. This has led to a provocative discussion of whether homone therapy should be instituted after menopause to protect against heart disease. On the face of it, it would seem a good idea (hormone therapy would also reduce the "hot flashes" associated with menopause). What complicates the issue is whether or not such hormone therapy can increase breast and uterine cancer rates. Although the final word is not yet in on this subject, the American College of Physicians issued guidelines in 1992 to help physicians counsel postmenopausal women about preventive hormone therapy. Based on a mega-review of the effects of estrogen therapy—and estrogen plus progestin therapy—on heart disease and cancer, the guidelines are as follows:

1. All women, regardless of race, should consider preventive hormone therapy.

2. Women who have had a hysterectomy are likely to benefit from estrogen therapy. There is no reason to add a progestin to the hormone regimen in such women.

3. Women who have coronary heart disease are likely to benefit from hormone therapy. If such women have a uterus, progestin should not be added to the estrogen therapy unless careful endometrial monitoring is performed.

4. The risks of hormone therapy may outweigh its benefits in women who are at increased risk for breast cancer.

5. For other women, the best course of action is not clear.

Aside from these recommendations to the postmenopausal woman, what other advice can we offer? First and foremost—do not smoke (see Chapter 7). Secondly, reduce your intake of animal fat. Thirdly, get plenty of aerobic exercise, and keep an eye on your blood pressure. If this sounds similar to the advice we give men, it should be because it is the same! Women do have one special worry, however. The combination of birth-control pills and smoking seems to lead to development of blood clots in both the arteries and veins. Even young women are at risk. Women also have another special problem. Because their body size is smaller than men, their blood vessels are smaller (narrower). Therefore, blockages of the same absolute size are more serious in women since the vessel channel is narrower from the beginning. This makes surgery and angioplasty more difficult and emphasizes the need for effective preventive measures and early diagnosis.

CHAPTER
— 14 —

Older Hearts:
Heart Disease
over the Age of 65

In general, older persons with heart disease are treated the same way as younger people. The major caveat concerns drugs, which must be more carefully regulated. In addition, a different set of psychological concerns occupies individuals who are in their retirement years and have heart disease. As far as preventing heart disease in older persons who don't already have it, the same attention to risk factor control is advised, but exercise programs must accentuate activities such as walking that cause less trauma to their more fragile bone structure.

On a recent winter vacation in Florida, we frequently found ourselves in the company of ex-Northerners who had retired to the South. When we discussed the content of this book with them, they seemed as interested as other, younger people with whom we had talked, but they also had questions about heart disease that they felt were of special concern to older people and wondered if these questions would be answered by reading the book. Upon reflection, we thought the best way to address these concerns would be in a separate chapter with a different kind of format—one that used a direct question and answer approach to the problems of the "older heart."

1. *Is silent heart disease more common in older people?*

Yes. Using a working definition of 65 as the beginning of old age (because it is a common retirement age), several studies especially the Baltimore Longitudinal Aging Study, have shown that silent heart attacks are more common in the older population. The reasons are twofold: Structural changes occur in the nerve tissue that transmits pain sensations from the heart, and there is diminished recognition of pain by higher centers in the brain. Older people who are often forgetful may simply not remember brief episodes of chest discomfort that later on routine electrocardiograms turn out to have been a heart attack. Whether older persons also have more frequent episodes of silent myocardial ischemia is not known at this time.

2. *Are risk factors as important in older people?*

Yes. While it is true that increasing age is an important factor in the development of coronary artery blockage, cigarette smoking, high blood pressure and high serum cholesterol can accelerate this process in older people. Data from the Framingham Study show that these risk factors are important—regardless of age—in causing heart disease. Once heart disease develops, they are still important, just as with younger people.

3. *Should older people have annual exercise tests?*

Routine screening in this generally less active age group is not recommended, but if a patient has angina, or has had a heart attack, the exercise test can still provide important prognostic information.

4. *Is coronary arteriography more dangerous in older persons?*
No.

5. Is stress less of a factor in causing heart disease in this age group?

Probably. The demands of the workplace are no longer a problem, and this alone removes a great deal of stress. Similarly, the most difficult child-raising years are long gone; though parent–child relationships can still cause one's temper to rise from time to time.

6. Once older persons have heart disease, how does this affect their life span?

The major prognostic features are still the extent of coronary artery disease and the ability of the left ventricle to pump blood normally. Age itself does not enter into the equation. Of course, other serious diseases that are commonly present in the older population (kidney disease, lung disease, cancer) can shorten the life span.

7. How vigorous should risk-factor correction be in older people?

Cigarette smoking is always bad, period.

Treating high blood pressure too vigorously can present problems. Because the stiffer blood vessels of the older person's brain and kidney require a higher driving (systolic) pressure, physicians do not attempt to lower blood pressure to the same levels as they do with younger persons. To do so may result in unacceptable side effects from either the lower pressure itself or the high doses of drugs needed to reach that level. Thus, a goal of 150/90 mm may be entirely reasonable in a 70-year-old with a blood pressure of 180/100, whereas in a 40-year-old the goal would be 120/80. For elderly black patients, however, the physician tries to walk a middle road because of the high incidence of strokes due to high blood pressure in this group.

Cholesterol lowering in the older age group is controversial since plaque formation takes years to develop. Using the kinds of recipes provided in this book will certainly cause no harm, but pushing drugs with uncomfortable side effects may cause the patient more harm than good.

8. *Does the more fragile bone structure of older people make exercise more dangerous?*

For certain activities, yes, but not for walking and bicycling. These are recommended for persons free of heart disease, but they must be carefully regulated in persons with known heart disease. We do not recommend that anyone, young or old, exercises to the point of pain.

9. *Are there special precautions to be aware of in prescibing medications for the over-65 population?*

Yes, particularly with the beta blockers. These drugs slow the heart rate, and because older patients are more prone to develop very slow heart rates on normal dosage, physicians must be extremely careful. That is not to say the drugs cannot be used— they can be, but extra care must go into determining the dosage schedule. Nitrates and calcium blockers may lead to more light-headedness and dizziness in older people because of a tendency for blood pressure to fall temporarily when they stand up. This reaction is true of any of the anti-hypertensive drugs.

10. *Are balloon angioplasty and coronary surgery still viable options in older patients?*

Definitely. Several studies have shown that coronary artery surgery can be performed with low risk in patients in their 70s whose symptoms or anatomy indicate that surgery will be helpful. The risks of balloon angioplasty are also not greatly different in this age group. It is especially useful in older people with other diseases (such as lung or kidney problems) that make their coronary surgery risky. Here, balloon angioplasty can truly be a lifesaver.

11. *Does the revolution in heart attack treatment also apply to the elderly?*

Yes and no. Older people have a greater risk of intracranial bleeding (which can cause a stroke) when clot-dissolving drugs are given into veins. Fortunately, this undesirable side effect is only seen in about 1% of patients. All other advances in heart attack care can be applied to the elderly, though again the dosage of cardiac drugs has to be more carefully controlled.

12. *Do older patients with heart disease have unique sexual problems?*

Not really. Younger people often assume that those over 65 do not, or should not, engage in an active sexual life. In reality, there is no reason why anyone with heart disease who has recovered to a point where he or she is able to climb stairs and resume other normal activities cannot resume his or her usual sexual activities. Some couples find that a less physically active sexual life, including masturbation and/or oral sex, makes them feel more secure. After the afflicted person has had an orgasm without any angina or discomfort, the couple usually resumes their previous sexual routine. Rarely do couples have a more satisfying sexual life after the onset of heart disease, but indeed there is no reason why they cannot.

13. *What are the common psychological problems in people over 65 years of age with heart disease?*

Retired people with heart disease often face different problems than their younger counterparts, especially when they are recovering from heart attacks. Those who have led active lives often have problems adjusting to the more sedentary retirement life. Women must learn to cope with having their husbands home more often and their time becomes more constricted. They don't have the freedom to work, shop or play without feeling guilty for leaving their mate at home. Consequently, when a spouse is afflicted with heart disease, his or her recovery can become more difficult. Men often have a tendency to become cardiac cripples; they can now justify a less active existence, and their spouses can resume their previous roles of primary care-giver in the home. These couples may need psychological help so that they can both lead a more productive life.

When both members of a couple have worked outside the home and have another life independent from one another, the recovery may be easier. Each person has had the experience of enjoying a separate existence during the day. Consequently, when the heart patient has recovered sufficiently, the couple can continue to enjoy their previous life without the mutual "need" to create a cardiac cripple.

14. *What problems do older people face when their child suffers from heart disease?*

When the child of an older couple has heart disease, the parents often feel guilty, wondering what they have done wrong. Parents usually feel more comfortable when they themselves suffer rather than their children. Often older people may have to help in the care of their grandchildren when their child or in-law has a heart attack. Extended stays in someone else's home, especially when a medical crisis has happened, can be very difficult. Responsibilities such as changing diapers or driving carpools that have long been left behind must become a part of everyday life again.

15. *Aren't there also different economic problems in the elderly that can affect their living with heart disease?*

Because so many people in this age group are retired or are married to people who are, the concerns about returning to work are obviously far fewer. On the other hand, fear of prolonged hospitalization or of transfer to a nursing home can be great. These fears are compounded by the realization that medical and nursing care are expensive. This is especially true outside the hospital when the insurance coverage is not usually as extensive. Coupled with the medications themselves, the burden of heart disease or any other major illness can prove catastrophic for the older citizen living on retirement benefits. This is one of the great tragedies of our society. With luck, advances in medical care will not only include scientific breakthroughs but also new laws to more fully protect our older population from the economic ravages of chronic disease.

CHAPTER

15

What's Next?

In the future, the key to fighting heart disease will still be in prevention. New techniques to identify people at risk and to detect silent heart disease before a fatal event occurs are already close to reality. The treatment phase will emphasize new drugs to reduce cholesterol levels and more innovative approaches to eliminating clots and fatty deposits in diseased coronary arteries.

Predicting the future is never easy, but in cardiology there are some early reports that, if true, are bound to change the way we think of heart disease.

For example, the entire field of prevention could be made more palatable to all of us if we knew in advance who among us were most susceptible to heart disease in later life. It is true that our family histories and our risk-factor profiles provide valuable data in this regard. Early results of studies in offspring of adults with heart disease have shown that some offspring already have higher blood pressure and cholesterol levels than do their peers, or even than some of their siblings. These children require aggressive risk-factor management. To identify these children, more intensive screening of the children of parents with heart disease is needed. This may involve isolation of genes in the search for even more sophisticated "markers" of future disease.

Prevention will also be greatly enhanced when the public finally realizes that all of the admonitions about cigarette smoking are true. They are not empty threats. Cigarette smoking is Russian roulette, pure and simple. The great gains we have made in treating hypertension, and lowering the animal fat and cholesterol consumption in our diets, will soon reach a plateau if cigarette smoking does not decrease further.

We have emphasized that detection of heart disease, before the symptomatic phase begins, relies on exercise testing and perhaps also Holter monitoring, as evidenced by a land-mark study from Sweden published in 1989. The education of physicians to screen their high-risk—but apparently healthy—populations must proceed at a faster pace. Future developments in Holter-related technology will make it easier to record episodes of daily ischemia in persons known to have heart disease. These devices will record "on-line" and will even be able to warn patients (via a buzzer) when ischemia or arrhythmias are occurring! The patient will then be able to take appropriate medications. In patients suspected of having heart disease, new imaging technology will allow blockages to be visualized without the need for coronary arteriography!

What about the treatment of heart disease? We have repeatedly stressed that one ounce of prevention is worth a pound of cure. But until the public accepts the lifestyle changes that we and others urge them to accept, heart disease will continue to be the number one killer, and advances in treatment will continue to be important. We foresee a significant increase in the number of balloon angioplasties being performed, with the greatest increase in patients admitted with acute heart attacks. Refinements in this technique are constantly being tested in animals and humans. In addition to these studies, others are examining why a given plaque becomes "active," that is, a seeding area for clots. A leader in this field is Dr. Andrew Selwyn of the Harvard Medical School. "This plaque is not a fixed lesion. In some instances, constriction in the wall over the plaque makes the narrowing even more acute." Why does this happen? "It may be due to a 'roughening' of the lining cells, the endothelium. It is essential to learn more about this if we wish to treat it effectively."

Hand in hand with techniques to eliminate plaques will be those aimed at dissolving the clots that "sit" on the plaques and plug vital arteries to the heart muscle. In the next several years, every community hospital emergency room should be able to use intravenous injections of new, clot-specific dissolving agents. We hope this new class of agents will cause fewer generalized bleeding problems than does streptokinase or RT-PA. Genetic "manipulation" is also on the horizon, with vast ramifications.

Will all of these medical approaches cut down the need for surgery? Probably, but not to the extent some surgeons fear. There is simply too much disease out there to see much of a decline in the surgical cases. Along with medical and surgical advances will come a greater realization of the importance of strong family and social support for the patient—and we hope—a greater realization of the strain the patient's family is experiencing. Reduction of stress in our daily lives is probably not possible for most of us, but learning to cope with that stress is. Better living habits—including some type of whole-body exercise—are a must.

Finally, we think it is obvious that one of the "new" discoveries in heart disease, the importance of silent heart disease (the stimulus for this book!), will soon be accepted by physician and public alike. It is inconceivable that, after the advances in the 1970s and 1980s, we will ever again consider only a person's symptoms when we talk about heart disease. The importance of silent heart disease was recognized by the National Institutes of Health when it sponsored a workshop on the subject in 1986. Guidelines from that workshop were published in 1987 and should help physicians all over the country deal with this problem. This will be good for all of us because, in reality, the fight against this silent killer will play a large role in the fight against heart disease.

Glossary

ACE-inhibitor a type of heart drug used to treat high blood pressure and heart failure

angina discomfort due to coronary heart disease; includes pressure or pain in the chest, arms or jaw (also called *angina pectoris*)

angioplasty see *PTCA*

aorta main artery in the body

arrhythmia irregularity of the heartbeat

arteries blood vessels that carry blood from the heart to the rest of the body

atherosclerosis buildup of fatty deposits (plaques) in blood vessels

atrium thin-walled collecting chamber of the heart (left and right)

beta blocker a type of heart drug used mainly to treat angina and high blood pressure (also called *beta-adrenergic blocking agent*)

bypass surgery use of a vein to connect the aorta with an obstructed coronary artery (also called *coronary artery bypass surgery*)

calcium blockers a type of heart drug used to treat angina and high blood pressure (also called *calcium channel blocking agents* and *calcium antagonists*)

cardiac arrest cessation of the heartbeat

cardiac catheterization a procedure using special tubing (catheters) to study the heart's chambers and vessels

cholesterol an important fatty substance that the body uses in a variety of ways but one that can accumulate in arteries and block them when present in high levels in the blood. Most cholesterol in the body is made in the liver from saturated fats. The transport system for carrying cholesterol to and from the liver involves special protein compounds termed *lipoproteins*. Low density lipoproteins cause accumulation of cholesterol in vessel walls, while high density lipoproteins remove the cholesterol

contrast agent a dye used to inject blood vessels, heart chambers, etc. Prevents X-rays from passing through ("radio-opaque"), leaving the injected areas visible

coronary arteries arteries supplying blood to the muscular walls of the heart

coronary arteriogram that part of the cardiac catheterization procedure in which a contrast agent is injected into the coronary arteries and X-ray records are obtained

coronary artery disease heart disease (ischemia, infarction, arrhythmias, etc.) due to obstruction of blood flow in the coronary arteries (also called *coronary heart disease*)

coronary care unit (CCU) special part of hospital with intensive nursing care and equipment for heart disease patients

coronary risk factors factors (such as cigarette smoking) that predispose persons to the development of coronary heart disease

CPR abbreviation for *cardiopulmonary resuscitation*, a technique used to revive someone whose heart has stopped and who is not breathing

diabetes disease related to a high level of sugar in the blood (also called *diabetes mellitus*)

echocardiogram video or still frame recording of ultrasound waves that depict some of the structures of the heart

electrocardiogram recording of the electrical impulses of the heart (also called *ECG* or *EKG*)

Enhanced External Counter Pulsation (EECP) new device used to treat angina

exercise either aerobic (uses oxygen) or non-aerobic (uses other body fuel sources), either dynamic (with rhythmic movement of large muscle groups, like walking) or static (with muscle contraction and little movement, like weight lifting). A good physical conditioning program depends on aerobic, dynamic exercises

exercise test technique used to observe signs of ischemia and other heart problems. Person walks on treadmill while continuous electrocardiographic recording is obtained (also called *stress test*)

false-negative result test is normal (negative) but disease is present

false-positive result test is abnormal (positive) but no disease is present (as with false-positive exercise test)

fats these can be saturated, mono unsaturated or poly unsaturated. The degree of saturation refers to the chemical composition and particularly the ability to add hydrogen atoms. Saturated fats have no room in their chemical structure for additional hydrogen atoms (e.g., egg yolks and butter). Mono unsaturated fats can add 2 hydrogen atoms (e.g., olive and peanut oil) and polyunsaturated fats can add 4 (e.g., corn and safflower oil). Animal fats are mostly saturated fats and raise the cholesterol levels in the blood; vegetable fats (except for coconut and palm oils) are mostly unsaturated; they do not raise the cholesterol level and can reduce it

Framingham Study longitudinal study of health of residents in Framingham, Massachusetts, to determine risk factors for cardiovascular disease

gamma camera special X-ray camera that measures radioactive gamma particles and provides graphic images; used in cardiology for thallium stress tests and radionuclide ventriculograms

heart attack see *myocardial infarction*

heart failure buildup of fluid in body (especially feet and lungs) due to heart disease (also called *congestive heart failure*)

Holter monitor small device to record electrocardiogram for 24 hours or longer out-of-hospital

hypertension high blood pressure (over 140/90 mm mercury)

invasive procedure one in which the interior of the body is "invaded" either by catheters placed in large blood vessels, or by surgical or related procedures, e.g., angioplasty or insertion of an electronic pacemaker

infarction death of living cells because of insufficient blood supply (see also *myocardial infarction*)

ischemia temporary damage to living cells because of insufficient blood supply (see also *myocardial ischemia*)

lipoprotein the fat/protein complex that is used to transport cholesterol and related substances in the blood

myocardial infarction death of heart muscle due to insufficient blood supply, usually because of clot obstructing blood flow (lay term: *heart attack*)

myocardial ischemia temporary damage to heart muscle because of insufficient blood flow. When pain accompanies it, it is called *angina* or *angina pectoris*

nitrates type of heart drug used mainly to treat angina

non-invasive procedure one in which diagnostic instruments do not enter body, e.g., an electrocardiogram or echocardiogram

plaque fatty deposit in lining of blood vessel

psychosomatic illness related to psychological rather than physical causes, for example, nausea due to fear

PTCA abbreviation for *percutaneous transluminal coronary angioplasty*. An invasive procedure in which a special catheter with an inflatable balloon at one end is used to open blocked coronary arteries (also called *balloon angioplasty* or just *angioplasty*)

QRS complex a part of the electrocardiographic tracing related to the contraction (beating) of the ventricle

radionuclide procedure non-invasive test in which a very small amount of radioactive material (isotope) is injected into the body and its location in the heart detected by a gamma camera. An X-ray like picture of the heart is then created by a computer. Examples are the thallium stress test and the radionuclide ventriculogram

ST segment that part of the electrocardiographic tracing related to ventricular relaxation

silent heart disease painless myocardial infarction or myocardial ischemia

sudden death death within a short period of time after the person collapses unexpectedly (some physicians use a 1-hour period, others a 24-hour period)

thallium stress test exercise test in which a small amount of radioactive thallium is injected into a vein to help depict areas of the heart with a poor blood supply

thrombolysis dissolving a blood clot (thrombus) in a blood vessel

ventricle pumping chamber of the heart (left and right)

ventricular contraction pumping (beating) of the ventricle

ventricular fibrillation rapid, irregular and ineffective contractions of the ventricle. A fatal arrhythmia unless ended by an electric shock to the chest

ventricular relaxation filling of the ventricle with blood after it contracts

ventriculogram X-ray or X-ray-like picture of the beating heart. When obtained at cardiac catheterization, a contrast agent is used, when obtained non-invasively, a radioisotope is used (*radionuclide ventriculogram*)

Recipes
for Good Habits

This section is not specifically meant to be a cookbook. What we hope to accomplish is to give some guidelines for healthful cooking for both cardiac patients and for healthy individuals who would like to improve their chances of avoiding cardiovascular disease. Remember that strict dieting requires the supervision of a physician.

Neither of us claim to be a nutritionist or expert chef. We are health care professionals who know a good deal about nutrition and love to eat well. An important lesson to learn is that one can revise favorite recipes by doing the following:

1. Eliminate or reduce the amount of salt by at least one-half.
2. Cut the amount of sugar called for in half to start—and then add more, if necessary.
3. Change saturated fats to polyunsaturated ones—unsalted margarines taste very good for all cooking and baking products. Although butter and margarine have the same caloric value, the latter is probably more heart-healthy. Learn to use it in place of butter. The best margarines are those with a high

content of corn, safflower, sunflower or soybean oil. Soft margarines are better than hard.

4. Cut down the amount of oil or margarine used in cooking. Most recipes call for much too much fat. Some recipes that call for sautéing don't need that step at all if the food is being added to a spicy casserole. If the ingredients need to be sautéed try water with a touch of oil.
5. Substitute low-fat yogurt for sour cream.
6. Cut down on high sodium products, such as soy sauce in Oriental cooking—one can sauté or stir-fry with water, adding low sodium soy sauce for taste.
7. Try the many delicious non-fat products now available.

Making meals interesting day after day, week after week, month after month, year after year, is a challenge for any meal planner and cook. The recipes that follow were selected to provide ideas for variety. In addition to these recipes provided, we suggest baking, broiling or barbecuing chicken, fish, lean cuts of lamb, beef and veal. One of our favorite meals consist of marinating chicken and grilling it outside on the gas grill. Broiling or barbecuing is a natural way of decreasing the amount of fat because the juices are left in the bottom of the pan or grill. Two favorite ways of serving vegetables are to steam them until they are crunchy and serve them "au naturel" or grill them on the barbecue with little or no oil. There is no need for any additions because vegetables are tasty by themselves. A simple but wonderful meal might include broiled fresh salmon, sprinkled with lemon and crushed garlic, steamed asparagus, boiled small new potatoes and fresh strawberries.

Each menu has dishes that can be used for family or company meals. None of the recipes are difficult. Only the yeast bread is time consuming.

In order to cut down the amount of fat that you consume, we suggest that you purchase three special things for your kitchen. Treat yourself to a large coated frying pan, either T-Fal or Silverstone. Non-stick coatings on kitchenware have been perfected over the years; the pans used presently do not chip. By using this kind of pan, you can reduce your use of oils or margarine, to a minimum. Also purchase a can of vegetable cooking spray such as Pam or Mazola No-Stick, which is especially helpful in baking when you need to grease a pan. When we refer to "greasing" in our recipes, it means to spray the container with a vegetable spray. We also suggest that you buy a gravy-grease separating container. They come in both a small and large size. When pan juices, soups and broths are poured into this container, it separates the liquid and the fat. You can then use the fluid to serve with your food after the fat has been thrown away.

A chicken stock recipe is included in the recipes because chicken broth is used in many recipes (see Mushroom Soup recipe on Monday night). If you use bouillon, use a low sodium product.

As mentioned in Chapter 8, the American Heart Association has issued new guidelines suggesting that only 30% of our daily consumption of food consist of fat. They also state that we only need to consume approximately 6–8 ounces of protein and no more than 3 grams of sodium per day. What this means is that we need to re-think our way of eating. Consume less meat, poultry and fish, and eat more vegetables, pasta, grains and bread.

We have included delicious and interesting heart-healthy desserts for each night of the week. However, there is no need to have dessert; it is only a complement to a meal. If you do choose to have cookies or cakes, have only two or three small cookies or one slice ($\frac{1}{16}$) of cake or sweet bread.

There are different ways to use these menus. You can follow them as they are, which will provide a heart-healthy, nutritious and filling meal. You can switch the vegetables, main courses or desserts from one night to another. Another suggestion is to grill a piece of chicken or fish, and serve it with one of the salads, potatoes and desserts suggested.

All of these recipes have been tested in our kitchen and approved for taste and appearance by ourselves and our sons. They have also been reviewed by a registered dietician. Enjoy eating and stay heart-healthy.

Vegetarian Chili
Brown Rice
or
Pita Bread
Oatmeal Cookies
or
Fresh Pineapple

Vegetarian Chili

8 servings

2   tablespoons olive oil
2   medium onions, chopped coarsely
4   cloves garlic, minced
2   large green peppers, cored, seeded and diced into ¼-inch pieces
1   can (28–35 ounces) unsalted tomatoes
1   medium eggplant, unpeeled, cut into ½-inch cubes
1½ pounds (approximately 10) plum tomatoes cut into 1-inch cubes
1   tablespoon chili powder
1   teaspoon ground cumin
1   tablespoon dried oregano (⅛ cup fresh, chopped)
1   tablespoon dried basil (¼ cup fresh, chopped)
1–2 teaspoons freshly ground pepper
1   teaspoon fennel seeds
2   tablespoons dried parsley (½ cup fresh, chopped)
1   can dark red kidney beans, drained
1   can chick-peas, drained

½ cup chopped fresh dill
2 tablespoons lemon juice
Brown rice (optional)
Low-fat cheddar cheese (optional)
Pita bread (optional)

1. Heat 2 tablespoons of oil in a skillet. Add onions, garlic, and green peppers and sauté just until softened, about 5 minutes. Put in a large pot.

2. Place the pot over low heat. Add eggplant, canned tomatoes with their liquid, fresh tomatoes, chili powder, cumin, oregano, basil, pepper, fennel and parsley. Cook uncovered, stirring frequently, for 30 minutes.

3. Stir in kidney beans, chick-peas, dill and lemon juice and cook another 15 minutes.

4. Serve immediately alone, or with brown rice and/or cheddar cheese. Can be eaten cold in pita bread as sandwiches.

Brown Rice
4-6 servings

2 cups brown rice
4 cups water

1. Cover the rice with the water and allow to sit in cooking pot for a minimum of 2 hours before cooking (can be overnight).

2. Bring water and rice to a boil, reduce heat and simmer rice in covered pot until water has been absorbed, about 15–20 minutes.

Oatmeal Cookies

60 cookies

¾	cup unsalted margarine
¾	cup dark brown sugar
¼	cup granulated sugar
1	egg or egg substitute
¼	cup water
1	teaspoon vanilla extract
3	cups uncooked oatmeal
1¼	cups flour
½	teaspoon salt
½	teaspoon baking soda
½	cup raisins (optional)
½	cup nuts (optional)

1. Preheat oven to 350°F.

2. Beat together margarine, sugars, egg, water and vanilla until creamy.

3. Combine oatmeal, flour, salt and baking soda.

4. Mix wet and dry ingredients well. Add raisins or nuts, if desired.

5. Drop by rounded teaspoonfuls onto a cookie sheet.

6. Bake at 350°F 12–15 minutes.

Fresh Pineapple

4 servings

1. Cut a pineapple into four pieces.

2. Remove the tough inner core.

3. Cut pineapple quarters lengthwise and into ½-inch slices across.

4. Chill and serve.

Fresh Mushroom Soup
Pan-Blackened Fish (Cajun Style)
Steamed Broccoli
Roasted Potatoes
Chocolate Meringue Drops
or
Baked Bananas

Fresh Mushroom Soup

4–6 servings

2	cups hot chicken stock or broth (recipe on page 203)
2–3	cloves garlic
12	ounces fresh mushrooms, sliced
4	tablespoons flour
2	cups skimmed milk
3	tablespoons finely chopped fresh parsley
	Grated nutmeg to taste
	Fresh pepper to taste
3	tablespoons dry sherry (optional)

1. Sauté garlic and mushrooms in 4 tablespoons of the chicken stock. Cook on very low heat, stirring constantly for 4 minutes. Remove mushrooms.

2. Put 2 tablespoons of flour into the saucepan. Add ½ cup chicken stock, additional flour, and slowly add the remaining chicken stock, stirring constantly. Add the milk. Return mushrooms to pan.

3. Bring to a boil, stirring continuously. Turn heat down and simmer for 5 minutes.

4. Add nutmeg, parsley and pepper. Add sherry, if desired. May be prepared a day ahead.

Pan-Blackened Fish *(Cajun Style)*
4-6 servings

Cajun Spice Mixture
1   teaspoon garlic
½   teaspoon onion powder
1   teaspoon black pepper
1   teaspoon red pepper (cayenne)
½   teaspoon dried thyme
½   teaspoon dried oregano

1   tablespoon corn or safflower oil
¼   cup safflower or corn oil margarine, melted
4   ½-inch thick fillets of salmon (approximately 4–6 ounces per person)
    Lemon wedges for serving

1. Combine the ingredients for the spice mixture.

2. Heat a dry cast-iron frying pan wiped with oil over high-heat setting until it turns a white/bluish-grey color, 10–15 minutes.

3. Meanwhile, brush a few tablespoons of margarine on each fish fillet. Sprinkle the fillets with spice mixture. They should be evenly coated but not too thickly crusted. Coat the other side with the remaining margarine and spices.

4. Put the fish into the frying pan and cook 4 minutes. Turn and cook 4 minutes on the other side.

5. Don't be upset by all the smoke. The fish should be singed but not burned.

6. Transfer the fish to warm plates and garnish with lemon wedges.

Steamed Broccoli

4–6 servings

1 Wash a head of broccoli well and drain. Remove the large coarse leaves and cut off the tough lower ends of the stalk.
2 Cut broccoli either lengthwise or in half.
3 Steam in about 1 inch of water 10–15 minutes.

Roasted Potatoes

4–6 servings

4 baking potatoes
1 tablespoon olive oil
   No-salt spices (e.g., Mrs. Dash, American Heart Association spice) (optional)

1. Preheat oven to 425°F.

2. Cut potatoes crosswise into rounds or cut into eighths lengthwise.

3. Brush with olive oil.

4. Bake at 425°F 15–20 minutes. Turn; bake 15–20 minutes or until brown.

5. Sprinkle with spices, if desired. An alternative is to add both whole garlic cloves and/or crushed garlic before basting potatoes.

Chocolate Meringue Drops

35 small cookies

2 egg whites
⅔ cup sugar
2 tablespoons cocoa
1 teaspoon vanilla extract
¾ cup walnuts, chopped (optional)

1. Preheat oven to 350°F.

2. Beat egg whites until they are stiff but not dry.

3. Combine sugar and cocoa.

4. Beat sugar and cocoa mixture into the egg whites, one tablespoon at a time.

5. Add vanilla.

6. Add walnuts, if desired.

7. Drop by teaspoonfuls onto greased and lightly floured cookie sheet.

8. Bake at 350°F for 10 minutes.

9. Allow to cool for 1 minute before removing from pan.

Baked Bananas

4-6 servings

4 large, ripe bananas
½ cup water
¼ cup packed brown sugar

1. Preheat oven to 375°F.
2. Slice bananas in half lengthwise and place in a shallow ovenproof pan.
3. Mix water and brown sugar in saucepan. Cook 5 minutes.
4. Put brown sugar syrup on bananas.
5. Cook in a 375°F oven for 15 minutes. Turn and baste with syrup and cook 15 minutes more.

Chicken Broth

9 cups

1	3 pound chicken (or 2–3 pounds backs and wings)
3	quarts water (12 cups)
2	medium onions, peeled and cut in quarters
3	carrots, peeled and cut in quarters
2	teaspoons salt
1	teaspoon freshly ground pepper
4	ribs celery with leafy tops or 3 celery stalks
2	bay leaves
1	teaspoon dried thyme (1 fresh sprig)
1	teaspoon dried parsley (3 parsley sprigs)
3	parsnips (optional)

1. Combine all ingredients in a large pot.
2. Bring to a boil, reduce heat and simmer 2–3 hours.
3. Skim off fat and froth as it is cooking.
4. Remove chicken from pot and save for another use.
5. Strain stock through a fine mesh sieve into a clean saucepan. Discard the solids. Let the stock cool. Skim off any fat from the top.
6. Refrigerate overnight and skim again. Can be frozen for future use.

Zucchini Soup
Baked Chicken Breasts with Mushrooms and Grapes
Steamed Green Beans
Brown Rice (recipe on page 197)
Angel Food Cake
or
Fresh Fruit Compote

Zucchini Soup
4–6 servings

6   medium zucchini, cut in pieces (approximately 1-inch rounds)
2   medium large onions, coarsely chopped
2   cloves garlic, crushed
4   cups chicken or vegetable broth (recipe on page 203)
⅓   cup fresh basil, chopped

1. Place zucchini, onions, garlic and broth in a saucepan.

2. Bring to a boil, cover and simmer 35 minutes.

3. Add basil.

4. Put mixture into a food processor or blender. Puree.

5. Serve warm or chilled.

Baked Chicken Breasts with Mushrooms and Grapes

4–6 servings

4	chicken breasts, split, skinned and boned
	Pepper to taste
¼	cup onions, chopped
½	cup chicken broth (recipe on page 203) (reserve 4 tablespoons)
½	cup dry white wine
½	pound fresh mushrooms sliced (2 cups)
¼	pound seedless grapes (2 cups)

1. Preheat oven to 350°F.

2. Arrange breasts together in a shallow pan. Sprinkle with pepper.

3. Combine chicken broth and wine in saucepan. Add onions. Bring to a boil.

4. Pour sauce over the chicken.

5. Cover and bake 1 hour.

6. Cook mushrooms in reserved broth for 1–2 minutes.

7. Add to chicken along with grapes.

8. Cover and continue to bake for 10 minutes or until grapes are just heated.

Steamed Green Beans

4–6 servings

1½   pounds green beans
     Water

1. Remove ends and strings from the beans. Leave whole, snap in half or cut into thin, lengthwise strips.

2. Steam in 1 inch of boiling water 8–10 minutes until barely tender.

3. Strain and serve.

Angel Food Cake

16 servings

1¼   cups sugar
 1   cup cake flour[1]
 ¼   teaspoon salt
12   egg whites, room temperature
 1   teaspoon cream of tartar
 1   teaspoon flavoring[2]

1. Preheat oven to 350°F.

2. Sift sugar two times.

3. Sift flour before measuring.

4. Sift ¼ cup of the sugar with the flour and the salt three times.

5. Beat egg whites until foamy. Add the cream of tartar and beat until stiff, not dry. Beat in the flavoring.

6. Beat in the remaining sugar 1 tablespoon at a time.

7. Add flavoring and beat again until the peaks are stiff and glossy.[3]

8. Gently fold flour mixture into egg white mixture.

9. Pour batter into ungreased 10-inch tube pan. Bake 45–50 minutes or until cake springs back when touched.

10. Remove the pan from the oven and turn it upside down over the top of a wine or soft drink bottle to cool for at least 2 hours.

11. Run a knife around the sides of the pan before you try to remove it.

12. Serve with chocolate sauce, strawberries or plain.

[1] Variation for Chocolate Angel Food Cake. Use ¾ cup flour and ¼ cup cocoa sifted in place of 1 cup flour.

[2] Use a total of 1 teaspoon flavoring: that can be 1 teaspoon vanilla extract, ½ teaspoon vanilla and ½ teaspoon almond extract, 1 teaspoon almond extract, or ½ teaspoon maple flavoring and ½ teaspoon vanilla extract.

[3] At this point you can make additions to the recipe. For example: ½ cup chopped walnuts, 1 cup unsweetened canned fruit (drained), 1 teaspoon cinnamon, ½ teaspoon nutmeg or ¼ teaspoon cloves.

Fresh Fruit Compote
4–6 servings

1	orange, peeled and cut into sections
1	apple, peeled and cut into bite-size pieces
1	grapefuit, peeled and cut into sections
½	cup strawberries, cleaned and hulled
½	cup raspberries, cleaned
½	cup grapes
1	kiwi, peeled and sliced
1	banana, peeled and sliced
¼	pineapple
3	tablespoons kirsch or framboise (optional)

1. Pick your favorite ripe fruits (these are just ideas).

2. Put them into a large glass bowl.

3. Toss with kirsch or framboise, if desired.

Linguine with Asparagus
Green Salad with Vinaigrette Dressing
French Whole-Wheat Bread
Raisin Cake
or
Melon (Honeydew, Cantaloupe, Watermelon, Cranshaw)

Linguine with Asparagus
4–6 servings

1½	pounds asparagus, cut on diagonal into ½-inch pieces
	Boiling water
¼	cup olive oil
3	large cloves garlic, crushed
4	medium tomatoes, chopped coarsely
4	large scallions, trimmed and cut into ⅛-inch slices
	Dash of crushed red pepper
	Freshly ground pepper to taste
1	pound linguine
1	cup coarsely chopped fresh basil
	Parmesan cheese (optional)

1. Put asparagus in a bowl. Cover with boiling water. Let sit for 3 minutes. Drain asparagus and save water.

2. Heat olive oil in a large skillet with garlic. Sauté about 2 minutes. Add tomatoes, scallions and both peppers. Cook about 4 minutes, stirring occasionally. Add asparagus and cook 1 minute to warm.

3. Put asparagus water (add additional water, if necessary) in large pot. Cook pasta *al dente*, according to directions.

4. Toss pasta into sauce and sprinkle with basil. Serve immediately. Sprinkle with grated Parmesan cheese, if desired.

Note: Cut-up broccoli, green beans or a variety of vegetables can be used in place of asparagus.

Green Salad with Vinaigrette Dressing

4–6 servings

Iceberg, romaine, bibb, Boston lettuce
¼ cup green onions or scallions
4 sprigs arugula (optional)
4 leaves endive (optional)
Vinaigrette dressing

1. Pick any of your favorite lettuce, wash, dry well and put into a salad bowl with the scallions.

2. Measure about 5 tablespoons of the salad dressing into the lettuce and toss.

Vinaigrette Dressing

1 cup

6 tablespoons Balsamic vinegar
1 tablespoon Dijon or imported grainy mustard
1 clove garlic, crushed
1 tablespoon water
6 tablespoons safflower oil

Mix all ingredients together in glass jar.

French Whole-Wheat Bread
1 loaf

1	package dry yeast (1 tablespoon)
1	teaspoon sugar
1½	cups warm water (105°–115°F)
2½	cups unbleached all purpose or bread flour
1¼	cups whole-wheat flour
½	teaspoon salt (optional)
2	tablespoons cornmeal
1	tablespoon water

1. Put water in a glass measuring container. Add yeast and sugar. Let stand 5–10 minutes until it bubbles.

2. Mix flours together. Add salt, if desired.

3. Put half the flour mixture in a bowl, add the yeast mixture and then the rest of the flour. Mix well.

4. Turn out on a floured surface, knead until smooth and elastic, about 8–10 minutes. Add additional flour as needed.

5. Place dough in a greased bowl and cover with waxed paper.

6. Let rise in warm place until doubled in size, about 40 minutes.

7. Punch down and turn out onto a floured surface. Knead for about 1 minute. Roll out dough to make a 15" x 10" rectangle. Roll up tightly on long side, like a jelly roll.

8. Place dough seam side down on a cookie sheet sprinkled with cornmeal. Place in a warm spot and allow to rise 30 minutes. Meanwhile, preheat oven to 400°F.

9. With a sharp knife or razor, make 3 diagonal cuts on top of loaves. Sprinkle with water and bake for about 30 minutes. (Bread should give a hollow sound when tapped.)

10. Allow to cool on rack before slicing.

Note: This bread is especially good toasted.

Raisin Cake

1 8-inch square pan

    1   cup raisins (muscat or Thompson)
    2   tablespoons unsalted margarine
    2   cups water
    ½   cup sugar
    1   teaspoon cinnamon
    ½   teaspoon ground cloves
    1   teaspoon baking soda
    2   cups flour
    ¼   teaspoon salt
    ½   cup walnuts (optional)

1. Preheat oven to 350°F.

2. Combine raisins, margarine, water, sugar, cinnamon and cloves; put in a saucepan and let simmer for 15 minutes. Let cool.

3. Sift 2 cups of flour with soda and salt.

4. Mix flour and spice mixtures. Add walnuts, if desired.

5. Pour into "greased" 8-inch square pan.

6. Bake in for 1 hour.

Melon

(Honeydew, Cantaloupe, Watermelon, Cranshaw)

Cut melon into slices appropriate for an individual serving or cut up a variety of melons and serve in a glass bowl. Garnish with a lemon slice.

Chicken with Vegetables and Potatoes
Date–Nut Bread
or
Baked Apples

Chicken with Vegetables and Potatoes
4–8 servings

  2 tablespoons olive oil
10 small white onions, peeled
  2 cloves garlic, crushed
½ pound mushrooms, sliced
  1 small eggplant, pared and cut into ½-inch strips
  1 teaspoon dried or ¼ cup fresh basil chopped
  1 green pepper cut into ¼-inch strips
  1 teaspoon freshly ground pepper
½ teaspoon dried or ¼ cup fresh thyme
  2 bay leaves
½ cup sherry
  2 2½–3½-pound chickens, cut into pieces
  6 large potatoes cut into eighths, parboiled
  4 medium tomatoes quartered or 12 cherry tomatoes
     Aluminum foil

Sauce

1. In a large T-fal or Silverstone frying pan, sauté onions and garlic in oil until they are golden.

2. Add sliced mushrooms, eggplant and green pepper. Sauté about 2 minutes.

3. Add seasonings, bay leaves and sherry.

Chicken

1. Preheat oven to 350°F.

2. Remove skin from the chicken. Place chicken and potatoes in 11 x 14-inch pan.

3. Pour sauce over chicken. Cover pan with aluminum foil and bake for 45 minutes.

4. Uncover, add tomatoes, cover again and bake 30 minutes longer.

Date–Nut Bread

1 large loaf

½	pound dates, chopped
1	cup boiling water
1	teaspoon baking soda
1	egg
¾	cup sugar
1½	tablespoons unsalted margarine
¼	teaspoon salt
1¾	cups flour
½	cup walnuts (optional)

1. Preheat oven to 325°F.

2. Combine dates, water and baking soda.

3. Beat sugar, egg, margarine, salt and flour. Add the liquid from the dates and beat until smooth.

4. Add dates and walnuts.

5. Bake for 1 hour.

Baked Apples

6 servings

6	medium baking apples (Rome, McIntosh)
1	teaspoon cinnamon
1	cup apple juice
1–2	cups water
	Raisins, walnuts (optional)

1. Preheat oven to 350°F.

2. Core apples.

3. Place apples in a shallow glass baking dish.

4. Fill holes in apples with apple juice and cinnamon. Raisins and nuts can be added, if desired.

5. Put water around apples.

6. Bake in a 350° oven for 1 hour.

Salad with Honey–Mustard Dressing
Cioppino (California Fish Stew)
Lemon Bread
or
Garlic Croutons
Dried Fruit Compote

Salad with Honey–Mustard Dressing

Bibb, romaine, red-leaf, Boston, iceberg lettuce
Endive
Arugula
Radicchio
Chicory

1. Select a variety of your favorite kinds of lettuce.

2. Measure about 5 tablespoons of the dressing into the greens and toss.

Honey-Mustard Dressing
1 cup

5   tablespoons safflower or olive oil
1   tablespoon honey
1   tablespoon Dijon mustard
4   tablespoons water
5   tablespoons raspberry-flavored vinegar

1. Mix all ingredients together in a small jar or bottle.

2. Chill.

Cioppino *(California Fish Stew)*
8–10 servings

1	stalk celery, sliced (1 cup)
2	medium onions, diced (1½ cups)
3	carrots, sliced (1 cup)
2	tablespoons olive oil
2	tablespoons water
½	cup fresh parsley, chopped
¼	cup celery leaves, chopped
2	cloves garlic, crushed
1	teaspoon dried rosemary
1	teaspoon dried sage
½	teaspoon dried thyme
½	teaspoon dried oregano
1	can (16 ounces) Italian plum tomatoes, unsalted
1	can (15 ounces) tomato sauce, unsalted
1	cup white wine
¾	teaspoon pepper
1	pound large shrimp, shelled and deveined
1	pound cod or halibut, cut into 2-inch squares
2	crabs without bodies or 1 cracked crab
16–20	scallops
16–20	fresh clams, scrubbed
1	cup green pepper, coarsely chopped
½	cup white wine (in addition to 1 cup added previously)
½	cup fresh parsley

1. Sauté celery, onions and carrots in 2 tablespoons olive oil and 2 tablespoons water in a 6-quart pot until golden. Add ½ cup parsley, celery leaves, garlic, rosemary, sage, thyme, oregano, tomatoes, tomato sauce, 1 cup of the wine and pepper. Heat to boil. Simmer until tomatoes are soft and sauce thickens.

2. Add shrimp, fish, crab, scallops, clams and green pepper. Simmer. Add the remaining ½ cup wine.

3. Sprinkle with ½ cup parsley before serving.

Note: One can include any combination of fish and seafood that is available.

Garlic Croutons for Cioppino

1   French bread (preferrably whole-wheat French bread)
     Garlic

1. Slice French bread into 1–1½-inch pieces.

2. Rub each side with a peeled garlic clove.

3. Bake in a 350°F oven until brown.

4. Serve with cioppino.

Lemon Bread

1 loaf

½   cup unsalted margarine
¾   cup sugar
1¼ cups unbleached white flour
1   teaspoon baking powder
¼   teaspoon salt
½   cup skimmed milk
½   cup finely chopped walnuts or pecans (optional)
    Grated rind of 1 lemon

Glaze

    Juice of 1 lemon
¼   cup sugar

Cake

1. Preheat oven to 350°F.

2. Cream margarine and sugar.

3. Sift together flour, baking powder and salt.

4. Add dry ingredients to creamed mixture, alternating with milk (end with dry ingredients).

5. Add nuts and lemon rind.

6. Pour into "greased" 9 x 5-inch loaf pan.

7. Bake 1 hour at 350°F.

Glaze

1. Mix lemon juice and sugar.

2. Remove bread from the pan after it has cooled for 15 minutes.

3. Immediately pierce surface of bread with a toothpick and pour glaze over it.

Dried Fruit Compote
4–8 servings

¼   pound raisins
¼   pound dried apricots
¼   pound dried apples
¼   pound dried peaches
¼   pound dried figs
¼   pound dried pears
    Water
    Zest of 1 lemon
2   cinnamon sticks

1. Dried fruit can be selected in any combination from a health food store or supermarket.

2. Cover fruits with water, add 2 cinnamon sticks and zest of lemon. Soak for ½ hour.

3. Simmer fruit about 15–30 minutes until tender.

4. Can be served warm or cold.

Cinnamon–Honey Chicken
Grated Zucchini
New Potatoes
Swedish Crescents
Strawberries with Raspberry Sauce

Cinnamon–Honey Chicken

4–8 servings

2   2½–3½-pound chickens, cut into pieces
½   cup dry sherry
1   tablespoon cinnamon
¼   cup honey
¼   cup lime or lemon juice
1   clove garlic, crushed
    Pepper to taste

1. Mix together sherry, cinnamon, honey, lime juice, garlic and pepper.

2. Remove skin from chicken.

3. Arrange chicken in a single layer in a shallow ovenproof pan. Pour marinade over chicken, turn pieces to coat well. Refrigerate overnight or longer; turn pieces occasionally.

4. Preheat oven to 350°F. Drain marinade and reserve. Cover chicken with aluminum foil; bake for 1 hour. Baste with marinade, turning once or twice.

Grated Zucchini
4-6 servings

3   medium zucchini
2   tablespoons margarine
1   clove garlic, crushed
   Grated nutmeg
   Pepper to taste

1. Grate unpeeled zucchini, set aside.

2. Heat margarine in a saucepan.

3. Saute garlic in margarine for 3 minutes, without browning.

4. Toss the zucchini into the hot garlic mixture and saute 2–3 minutes until tender.

5. Season with nutmeg and pepper. Serve immediately.

New Potatoes
4-6 servings

12   small new potatoes
   Water
2   tablespoons margarine (optional)
¼   cup fresh parsley, chopped (optional)
2   tablespoons fresh lemon juice (optional)

1. Scrub potatoes. Put in a pan and cover with water.

2. Steam in their jackets until just tender, about 10 minutes.

3. Optional: toss with margarine, parsley, and lemon juice.

Swedish Crescents
70 cookies

1 cup unsalted margarine
1 cup ground pecans or almonds
2½ cups flour, sifted
⅓ cup sugar
1 teaspoon vanilla extract
1 teaspoon almond extract
Confectioners sugar (optional)

1. Preheat oven to 350°F.

2. Combine all ingredients in the bowl of a mixer or food processor. Mix thoroughly.

3. Form pieces of dough into crescents, no larger than 2 inches tip-to-tip. Place on a baking sheet.

4. Bake at 350°F for 15–20 minutes until light brown.

5. Cool. Dust with confectioners sugar, if desired.

Strawberries with Raspberry Sauce
4–6 servings

1 pint strawberries
1 16-ounce package frozen raspberries
3 tablespoons sugar (optional)
1 tablespoon kirsch or framboise (optional)

1. Wash and hull strawberries.

2. Partially thaw raspberries and put in a blender or food processor. Add sugar and/or liquor, if desired.

3. Put strawberries into individual glass bowls or serving dish and spoon the raspberry puree over them.

4. Chill for at least 1 hour.

FIGHTING THE SILENT KILLER